Remember

Remember

The Science of Memory and the Art of Forgetting

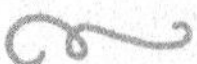

Lisa Genova

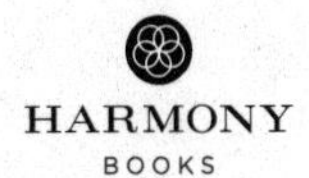

HARMONY
BOOKS

Published in the United States by Harmony Books,
an imprint of the Crown Publishing Group, a division of
Penguin Random House LLC, New York.
crownpublishing.com

Harmony Books is a registered trademark, and the Circle colophon
is a trademark of Penguin Random House LLC.

Library of Congress Cataloging-in-Publication Data
has been applied for.

ISBN 978-0-593-13795-6
ISBN 978-0-593-13796-3

Printed in the United States of America

Book design by Meighan Cavanaugh
Jacket design by Sarah Brody

10 9 8 7 6 5 4 3 2 1

First Edition

For Alena, Ethan, Stella, and Peanut

Contents

PART II

Why We Forget

PART III

Improve or Impair

Remember

Introduction

Picture a penny in your mind's eye. Because you've probably encountered a penny hundreds if not thousands of times over the years, you should have no trouble remembering what one looks like. You've committed this image to memory.

Or have you? Which president is pictured on the head of the penny? What direction is he facing? Are you sure? Where is the date? The words LIBERTY? IN GOD WE TRUST? What's pictured on the tail side? Could you draw both sides of a penny with total accuracy from memory right now? How can you both remember a penny and yet remember so little about it? Is your memory failing?

It's not. It's doing exactly what it's supposed to do.

Your brain is amazing. Every day, it performs a myriad miracles—it sees, hears, tastes, smells, and senses touch. It also feels pain, pleasure, temperature, stress, and a wide range of emotions. It plans things and solves problems. It knows where you are in space so you don't bump into walls or fall down when you step off a curb to cross the street. It comprehends and produces language. It mediates your desire for chocolate and sex, your ability to empathize with the joy and suffering of others, and an awareness of your own existence. And it can remember. Of all the complex and wondrous miracles that your brain executes, memory is king.

You need memory to learn anything. Without it, information and experiences can't be retained. New people would remain strangers. You wouldn't be able to remember the previous sentence by the end of this one. You depend on memory to call your mother later today and to take your heart medication before you go to bed tonight. You need memory to get dressed, brush your teeth, read these words, play tennis, and drive your car. You use your memory from the moment you wake up until the moment you go to sleep, and even then, your memory processes are busy at work.

The significant facts and moments of your life strung together create your life's narrative and identity. Memory allows you to have a sense of who you are and who you've been. If you've witnessed someone stripped bare of his or her personal history by Alzheimer's disease, you know firsthand how essential memory is to the experience of being human.

But for all its miraculous, necessary, and pervasive presence in our lives, memory is far from perfect. Our brains aren't designed to remember people's names, to do something later, or to catalog everything we encounter. These imperfections are simply the factory settings. Even in the smartest of heads, memory is fallible. A man famous for memorizing more than a hundred thousand digits of pi can also forget his wife's birthday or why he walked into his living room.

In fact, most of us will forget the majority of what we experience today by tomorrow. Added up, this means we actually don't remember most of our lives. How many days, in full, specific detail, can you remember from last year? Most people recall an average of only eight to ten. That's not even 3 percent of what you experienced from your recent past. You remember even less from five years ago.

And much of what we do remember is incomplete and inaccurate. Our memories for what happened are particularly vulnerable to omissions and unintentional editing. Do you remember where you were, who you were with, and what you were doing when President Kennedy was killed, when the space shuttle *Challenger* exploded, or when the Twin Towers collapsed on September 11, 2001? These recollections for shocking and emotional events feel vividly remembered even years later. But if you've ever reminisced about that day or read or watched a news report about it, then I'd bet every penny I've got that your confidently held, highly detailed memory is loaded with stuff you never actually experienced.

Accuracy aside, what does your brain remember?

Your first kiss
The answer to 6 × 6
How to tie your shoes
The day your son was born
The day your grandmother died
The colors of the rainbow
Your address
How to ride a bike

What does your brain most likely forget?

Your tenth kiss
What you had for dinner last Wednesday
Where you put your phone
The name of your fifth-grade teacher
The name of the woman you met five minutes ago
Algebra
To take out the trash
The Wi-Fi password

Why do we remember our first kiss but not our tenth? What determines what we remember and what we forget? Memory is quite economical. In a nutshell, our brains have evolved to remember what is meaningful. They forget what isn't. The truth is, much of our lives are habitual, routine, and inconsequential. We shower, brush our teeth, drink coffee, commute to work, do our jobs, eat lunch, commute home, eat dinner, watch TV, spend too much time on social media, and go to bed. Day after day. We can't remember anything about the load of laundry we did last week. And that's OK. Most of the time, forgetting isn't actually a problem to solve.

We would probably all agree that forgetting our tenth kiss, last week's laundry, what we ate for lunch on Wednesday, and whatever is on the head of a penny isn't such a big deal. These moments and details aren't particularly significant. However, our brains also forget plenty of things we do care about. I would very much like to remember to return my daughter's overdue library book, why I just walked into the kitchen, and where I put my glasses. These things matter to me. In these instances, we often forget not because it's efficient for our brains to do so but because we haven't supplied our brains with the kinds of input needed to support memory creation and retrieval. These garden-variety memory failures are normal outcomes of our brains' design. But we seldom think of them this way because most of us aren't familiar with our memory's owner's manual. We would remember more and forget less if we understood how the process works.

Most of what we forget is not a failure of character, a symptom of disease, or even a reasonable cause for fear—places most of us tend to go when memory fails us. We feel worried, embarrassed, or plain scared every time we forget something we believe we should remember or would have remembered back when we were younger. We hold on to the assumption that memory will weaken with age, betray us, and eventually leave us.

As both a neuroscientist and the author of *Still Alice,* I've been talking to audiences around the world about Alzheimer's disease and memory for over a decade. Without exception, after every speech, people wait for me in the lobby or corner me in the restroom to express their personal concerns about memory and forgetting. Many have a parent, a grandparent, or a spouse who had or has dementia. They have witnessed the devastation and the heartache caused by profound memory loss. When these folks can't remember their Netflix password or the name of that movie starring Tina Fey, they worry that these failures might be early signs that they, too, are succumbing to inevitable disease.

Our fears around forgetting aren't only about a dread of aging or Alzheimer's. They're also about losing *any* of our memory's capability. Because memory is so central to our functioning and identity, if you start becoming forgetful, if you begin forgetting words and start losing keys and glasses and your phone, the fear is this: *I might lose myself.* And that's justifiably terrifying.

Most of us paint forgetting as our mortal adversary, but it isn't always an obstacle to overcome. Effective remembering often requires forgetting. And just because memory sometimes fails doesn't mean it's in any way broken. While admittedly frustrating, forgetting is a normal part of being human. By understanding how memory functions, we can take these inconvenient gaffes in stride. We can also learn to prevent many episodes of forgetting by eliminating or artfully navigating around common errors and bad assumptions.

When I explain to folks why they forget things like names, where they parked their car, and whether they already took their vitamin today, when I describe how memory is created and retrieved and why we forget—not because of disease pathology but because of how our brains have evolved—they audibly exhale. They look relieved and grateful, changed by this information. They leave me unafraid, holding a new relationship with their memory. They are empowered.

Once we understand memory and become familiar with how it functions, its incredible strengths and maddening weaknesses, its natural vulnerabilities and potential superpowers, we can both vastly improve our ability to remember and feel less rattled when we inevitably forget. We can set educated expectations for our memory and create a better relationship with it. We don't have to fear it anymore. And *that* can be life changing.

While memory is king, it's also a bit of a dunce. There's a reason that you remember the words to every Beatles song and forget most of your own life or that you remember the Hamlet soliloquy you learned in tenth grade but forget what your spouse told you to pick up from the store five minutes ago. We both remember and forget what a penny looks like. Remembering pervades and facilitates everything we do. As does forgetting.

In this book, you'll learn how memories are made and how we retrieve them. Not all memories are created equal. There are many flavors—memories for the present moment, for how to do things, for the stuff you know, for what just happened, for what you intend to do later—and each memory is processed and organized in your brain in distinctly different ways. Some memories are built to exist for only a few seconds (a temporary passcode), whereas others can last a lifetime (your wedding day). Some are easier to create (your to-do list), others are easier to retrieve (what your daughter looks like), and still others are more likely to be forgotten (last Thursday's commute). You can depend on some kinds of memory to be highly accurate and reliable (how to drive your car). Others, much less so (everything that has happened).

You'll learn that attention is essential for creating a memory for anything. If you don't pay attention to where you park your car in the mall garage, you'll struggle to find it later, but not because you've forgotten where you parked. You have forgotten nothing. Without adding your attention, you never formed a memory for where you parked in the first place.

You'll learn whether forgotten memories are temporarily inaccessible, waiting to be unlocked with just the right cue (you can't remember a single word to "Bohemian Rhapsody" until someone else sings the first lyrics, and then you can belt out the entire song), or if they are erased forever (you remember nothing about the Peloponnesian War, no matter how many details are shared). You'll come to appreciate the very clear distinction between normal forgetting (you can't remember where you parked your Jeep) and forgetting because of Alzheimer's (you don't remember that you own a Jeep). You'll see how memory is profoundly impacted by meaning, emotion, sleep, stress, and context. And because of this, there are many things you can do to influence what your brain remembers and what it forgets.

Memory is the sum of what we remember and what we forget, and there is an art and science to both. Will you forget what you experience and learn today by tomorrow, or will you remember the details and lessons of today decades from now? Either way, your memory is miraculously powerful, highly fallible, and doing its job.

PART I

How We Remember

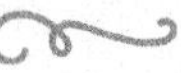

1

Making Memories 101

When Akira Haraguchi, a retired engineer from Japan, was sixty-nine years old—an age most of us associate with senior discounts and a less-than-optimal memory—he memorized pi, a nonrepeating, infinite number with no pattern, to 111,700 digits. That's the number 3.14159 . . . carried out to 111,695 more decimal places. From memory! If this sounds completely mind-blowing, I'm with you. Surely, you're thinking, Haraguchi must have been a child prodigy. Or perhaps he's a mathematical genius or a savant. He's none of these. He's a regular guy with a healthy, aging brain, which means something maybe even more mind-blowing—*your* brain is also capable of memorizing 111,700 digits of pi.

We can learn and remember anything—the unique sound of your child's voice, the face of a new friend, where you parked your car, that time you walked to the market all by yourself to buy sour cream when you were four years old, the words to the latest Taylor Swift song. The average adult has memorized the sound, spelling, and meaning of 20,000 to 100,000 words. Chess masters have memorized in the ballpark of 100,000 possible moves. Concert pianists who can play Rachmaninoff's third concerto have committed the coordination of almost 30,000 notes to memory. And these same folks don't need the sheet music to play Bach, Chopin, or Schumann, either.

Our memories can hold information that is deeply meaningful or nonsensical, simple or complex, and its capacity appears to be limitless. We can ask it to remember anything. And under the right conditions, it will.

How can memory do all of this? Neurologically speaking, what even is a memory? How is a memory made? Where are memories stored? And how do we retrieve them?

Making a memory literally changes your brain. Every memory you have is a result of a lasting physical alteration in your brain in response to what you experienced. You went from not knowing something to knowing something, from never before having experienced today to having lived another day. And to be able to remember tomorrow what happened today means that your brain has to change.

How does it change? First, the sensory, emotional, and

factual elements of what you experience are perceived through the portals of your senses. You see, hear, smell, taste, and feel.

Let's say it's the first evening of summer, and you're at your favorite beach with your best friends and their families. You see, among other things, your children playing soccer on the beach and a spectacular sunset glowing in the sky. You hear "Born This Way," one of your favorite Lady Gaga songs, playing over a portable speaker. Your daughter runs up to you, wailing, pointing to her bright pink ankle. A jellyfish has just stung her. Luckily, your friend carries a small container of meat tenderizer with her for this very scenario. You make a paste of the tenderizer and rub it on the sting, relieving your daughter's pain almost instantly (this really works). You smell the salty ocean air and smoke from the bonfire. You taste crisp, cold white wine, fresh briny oysters, and gooey sweet s'mores. You feel happy.

The sight of your children playing soccer has nothing to do with Lady Gaga or jellyfish or the taste of oysters, unless these fleeting, separate experiences become linked. To become a memory that you can later recall—*Remember that first night of summer, when we ate oysters and s'mores and listened to Lady Gaga while the kids played soccer on the beach and little Susie Q was stung by a jellyfish?*—all that previously unrelated neural activity becomes a connected pattern of neural activity. This pattern then persists through structural changes created between those neurons. The lasting change in neural architecture and connectivity can later be reexperienced—or remembered—through the activation of this now-linked neural circuit. This is memory.

Creating a memory takes place in four basic steps: *Encoding.* Your brain captures the sights, sounds, information, emotion, and meaning of what you perceived and paid attention to and translates all this into neurological language. *Consolidation.* Your brain links the previously unrelated collection of neural activity into a single pattern of associated connections. *Storage.* This pattern of activity is maintained over time through persistent structural and chemical changes in those neurons. *Retrieval.* You can now, through the activation of these associated connections, revisit, recall, know, and recognize what you learned and experienced.

All four steps have to work for you to create a long-term memory that can be consciously retrieved. You have to put the information into your brain. You have to weave the information together. You have to store that woven information via stable changes in your brain. And then you have to fetch the woven information when you want to access it.

How does a constellation of previously unrelated neural activity become bound together into a connected neural network that we experience as a singular memory? We're not entirely sure of how this happens, but we know a great deal about where it happens. The information contained within an experience that is collected by your brain—the sensory perceptions, the language, the who, what, where, when, and why—is linked by a part of your brain called the hippocampus.

The hippocampus, a seahorse-shaped structure deep in the middle of your brain, is essential for memory consolidation. What does that mean? The hippocampus binds your memories. It is your memory weaver. *What happened? Where and when did it happen? What does it mean? How did I feel about it?* The hippocampus links all these separate pieces of information from disparate parts of the brain together, knitting them into a retrievable unit of associated data, a neural network that, when stimulated, is experienced as a memory.

So your hippocampus is necessary for the formation of any new memories that you can later consciously retrieve. If your hippocampus is damaged, your ability to create new memories will be impaired. Alzheimer's disease begins its rampage in the hippocampus. As a result, the first symptoms of this disease are typically forgetting what happened earlier today or what someone just said a few minutes ago and repeating the same story or question over and over. With an impaired hippocampus, people with Alzheimer's have trouble creating new memories.

Moreover, the consolidation mediated by the hippocampus is a time-dependent process that can be disrupted. The formation of a memory that can be retrieved tomorrow, next week, or twenty years from now requires a series of molecular events that take time. During that time, if something interferes with the processing of a nascent memory in the hippocampus, the memory can be degraded and possibly lost.

Say you're a boxer, a football player, or a soccer player, and you sustain a blow to the head. If I were to interview you immediately after you got clocked, you would be able to tell me about the punch, the play, the details of what was happening. But if I were to ask you the next day, you might have no memory of what happened. The information that was in the process of becoming linked by your hippocampus to form a new, lasting memory was disrupted and was never fully consolidated. The blow to your head caused amnesia. Those memories are gone.

Damage to the hippocampus probably explains why Trevor Rees-Jones, bodyguard to Princess Diana and sole survivor of the car crash that killed her and Dodi Fyed all those years ago, still can't remember any details of what happened leading up to the accident. He sustained a devastating head injury, requiring many surgeries and about 150 pieces of titanium to reconstruct his face. Because the various elements of his pre-crash experience had not been fully linked together by his hippocampus when his brain was injured, they were never stored. Those memories of what happened were never made.

What happens if you don't have a hippocampus at all? Henry Molaison, or HM, as he is called in the thousands of papers citing his case for over half a century, is the most famous case study in the history of neuroscience. When Henry was a child, he fell off his bicycle, fracturing his skull. Whether because of this head injury or a family history of epilepsy no one is sure, but from the age of ten on, he regularly experienced debilitating seizures. Seventeen years later, his seizures still unrelenting and unresponsive to drug treatment, he was desperate and willing to try anything to get some relief. So on September 1, 1953, at the age of twenty-seven, Henry agreed to undergo experimental brain surgery.

The year 1953 was still well within the era of lobotomies and psychosurgeries, procedures that involved the indelicate removal or severing of brain regions to treat mental illnesses such as bipolar disorder and schizophrenia and brain disorders such as epilepsy. These kinds of surgical interventions are deemed grotesque, barbaric, and ineffective today, but back then, they were routinely performed by respected neurosurgeons. With the goal of eliminating Henry's seizures, a neurosurgeon named William Scoville removed the hippocampus and surrounding brain tissue from both sides of Henry's brain.

Here's the good news. Henry's seizures almost entirely subsided. And his personality, intelligence, language, motor function, and ability to perceive were undamaged by the procedure. So in that sense, the surgery was a success. But he had tragically traded one plague for another. The bad news was catastrophic. For the next fifty-five years until his death at the age of eighty-two, Henry could no longer consciously remember any new information or experience for more than a few moments. He would never again create a consciously held long-term memory.

He read the same magazines and watched the same movies over and over as if he had never seen them before. He greeted his doctor and the psychologists who studied him as if meeting them for the first time every single day. A Canadian psychologist named Brenda Milner studied Henry for more than fifty years, and in all that time, he never recognized her. He couldn't learn any new words. Vocabulary introduced to our lexicon after 1953—words like *granola*, *Jacuzzi*, *laptop*, and *emoji*—remained completely foreign to him. He could remember a number for a few minutes if he repeated it to himself over and over, but once he stopped rehearsing it, the number vanished forever. What's more, he would have no memory of having been asked to remember any number. He couldn't retain what happened minutes later, ever again.

So any new information from today that you perceive and attend to, that you find interesting, special, surprising, useful, meaningful, or, well, memorable, will be processed by your hippocampus for consolidation into memory. The hippocampus continues to repeatedly activate the parts of the brain involved in what-is-to-be-remembered until those parts of the brain become a stable, connected pattern of activity, essentially wired together.

While you need a hippocampus to form new memories, once they are made, they don't reside there. So where are memories stored? In no one place. They are distributed throughout the parts of the brain that registered the initial experience. Unlike perception and movement, which reside in specific addresses in our brains, we don't have specialized memory-storage neurons or a memory cortex. Vision, hearing, smell, touch, and movement can all be mapped to discrete geographic regions in the brain. At the back of the brain, we have a visual cortex, where neurons process what we see. We have an auditory cortex where we hear and an olfactory cortex where we perceive odor. Pain, temperature, and touch are housed in the somatosensory cortex on the top of your head. Wiggling your big toe can be mapped to the activation of a specific set of neurons in your motor cortex.

Memory is different. When we remember something, we're not withdrawing from a "memory bank." There is no memory bank. Long-term memories don't reside in one particular neighborhood in your brain.

Memory is stored throughout your brain in the pattern of neural activity that was stimulated when the event or information was first experienced. Your memory of last night's dinner requires the activation of the same constellation of disparate neurons that perceived, paid attention to, and processed your initial experience of that meal. Now, when some piece of the memory from last night's dinner is activated—someone asks you if you've ever eaten at Trattoria Il Panino in Boston's North End—the question triggers the activation of the connected network and you remember much, perhaps even all, about that time you ate there. *The weather was lovely, so my friend Tiff and I walked there. We had a conversational Italian lesson over dinner with John. I ate mushroom risotto. Delizioso!*

Memories physically exist in your head through a neural network of associations. My nana died of Alzheimer's in 2002. When I remember her, my brain is activating what she looked like in my visual cortex, the sound of her laugh in my auditory cortex, the smell of the sautéed green peppers and onions she cooked almost every day for lunch in my olfactory cortex, her red living room rug, the drums in the attic, the tin of *pizzelles* on the kitchen table, and so on.

Whenever we remember something, we are reactivating the various elements of the information we experienced, woven together as a single unit. Functional MRI brain imaging studies have glimpsed the act of retrieving a memory. When a person is asked to remember something while in an MRI scanner, we can literally see this person "searching his or her brain" for the information to be recalled. At first, brain activity flits around, lighting up all over the place. But when the pattern of activity in the brain matches the pattern of activity that occurred when the person first learned the information, it stabilizes there. And remarkably, it is then that the person will say, "I remember it!"

Similarly, the pattern of activation seen on a brain scan while someone is recalling a particular photograph is almost identical to the pattern of activation created when that person is physically looking at that photograph. Imagine Mickey Mouse. Got him? You "looked" inside your brain, and you can now "see" Mickey Mouse. The parts of your brain that are now activated include the same neurons in your visual cortex that would be activated if you were actually looking at a picture of Mickey Mouse. When imagining an image from memory, your brain is activated as if the image were right in front of you. To recall what you experienced or learned, your brain reactivates the elements of what you perceived and paid attention to in the first place.

Additionally, activating the memory of Mickey's image in your visual cortex might cause you to also remember other aspects of Mickey, say, the sound of his voice. So remembering Mickey Mouse might include what he looks like *and* what he sounds like. Activation of neurons in the visual cortex (what Mickey looks like) can trigger the activation of linked neurons that are distributed throughout the brain, which in this example includes neurons located in the auditory cortex (what Mickey sounds like). You can see and hear him.

But retrieval isn't like selecting an item on a DVD menu or a YouTube channel and pressing PLAY. We don't read our memories like a book or play them like a movie. Visual memory isn't like looking through your smartphone photo library, a collection of photos that can be zoomed in on and out of. You're not viewing a photograph. Remembering is an associative scavenger hunt, a reconstruction job that involves the

2

Pay Attention

Not long ago, somewhere in my midforties, I drove to Kendall Square in Cambridge, Massachusetts, from Cape Cod and parked my car in a garage. I checked the time and knew I had to hurry. I was scheduled to give a talk a couple of blocks away in a few minutes and had hoped to arrive sooner. Normally I take a photo of the floor number or the row letter as a record of my car's location whenever I park in a garage. But worried that I was going to be late, I raced out of there as fast as I could in heels without snapping a photo of my space and, worse, without consciously registering where I had parked.

I arrived on time, gave my forty-five-minute talk, answered

questions, and signed books. The whole affair probably took an hour and a half.

When I returned to the garage, I walked to where I thought I had parked, but my car wasn't there. I paced up and down ramps, becoming increasingly frustrated and hopeless as it remained missing. I walked from level to level, my feet screaming in my heels, sure I had parked on the fourth floor, but maybe it was the third or the fifth. And did I park in section A, B, or C? No idea. I couldn't remember. My car was nowhere. Gone.

I knew I was in the right garage, but that's all I had confidence in. I kept pressing the button on my car remote, trying not to panic, praying I would hear a beep-beep or see a flash of lights in response. Nothing. I was just about to report my car stolen when I stumbled upon it exactly where I left it, in 4B.

Relieved, embarrassed, and sweating, I reflexively wanted to blame the whole maddening experience on my memory, but the neuroscientist in me knew better. I couldn't find my car, not because I had a horrible memory, amnesia, dementia, or Alzheimer's. Temporarily losing my car had absolutely nothing to do with my memory.

I couldn't find my car, because I never paid attention to where I had parked it in the first place.

If we want to remember something, above all else, we need to notice what is going on. Noticing requires two things: perception (seeing, hearing, smelling, feeling) and attention. Let's say you're standing in front of the glitzy and colossal Christmas tree in Rockefeller Center in New York City. You take in the visual information—the shape, the size, the colors of the lights—through receptors called rods and cones in the retinas of your eyes. This information is converted into signals that travel to your visual cortex at the back of your brain, where the image is processed and actually seen. It can then be further processed in other brain regions for recognition, meaning, comparison, emotion, and opinion. But unless you add your attention to seeing this Christmas tree, the activated neurons will not be linked, and a memory will not be formed. You won't even remember seeing it.

Your memory isn't a video camera, recording a constant stream of every sight and sound you're exposed to. You can only capture and retain what you pay attention to. And since you can't pay attention to everything, you'll be able to remember some aspects of what is happening before you but not others. Think back to that first evening of summer on the beach. You remember the s'mores, the Lady Gaga song, and that Suzie Q was stung by a jellyfish. But surely there was more to see, hear, taste, and feel. Another parent there that night might remember hot dogs, beer, mosquitoes, and a seal sighting. You remember none of that. Your memories of the same evening are vastly different because of what you did and didn't pay attention to.

Think about the vast amount of information that your

senses are exposed to in any given day. If you're awake for sixteen hours today, your senses are open for business without a break for 57,600 seconds. That's a lot of data. But you simply can't and won't remember most of what was available to your eyes, ears, nose, and brain today.

Here's an example that will probably feel familiar. I frequently drive home to Cape Cod from Logan International Airport. About an hour into this trip and about forty minutes from home, I cross the Sagamore Bridge, a 1,408-foot, four-lane steel-arch bridge that spans the Cape Cod Canal. It's a formidable, memorable structure. At some point during this ride, I will typically and suddenly wonder, "Wait, did I already go over the bridge?" And then I'll notice that I'm at exit 5 on Route 6, which means I crossed the canal about ten minutes ago. I'm on Cape Cod and have *no* memory of having driven over that enormous bridge.

But surely my eyes saw it. The visual information was perceived by my eyes, and the image of the bridge made its way into the visual cortex in my brain. My brain definitely saw the bridge. And it's not as if I'm now asking my brain to recall some obscure detail I experienced from childhood. I drove over the bridge only ten minutes ago!

But I can't recall it, because this memory was never created in the first place. It's not enough for my senses to perceive information. My hippocampus can't consolidate any sensory information into a lasting memory without the neural input of attention. So because I wasn't paying attention to the bridge, the experience of driving over it slipped out of my brain within seconds, gone without a trace.

The number one reason for forgetting what you just said, a person's name, where you put your phone, and whether you already drove over a really big bridge is lack of attention. You can't later remember what is right in front of you if you don't pay attention to it. For example, if you don't notice where you put your glasses, you can't form a memory of where you put them. Later, when you're frustrated, unable to find them, you're not experiencing a true memory failure. You haven't forgotten anything, because the memory was never formed. Your glasses are missing because of a lack of attention (they're usually on my head!).

So if we want to remember something, we first have to pay attention to it. Unfortunately, this isn't so simple. Even if we didn't live in such a highly distractible time, paying attention isn't easy for our brains. In driving over the Sagamore Bridge, for example, I might have been distracted by a conversation or some delicious daydream, my attention diverted. More likely, I didn't register driving over the bridge because that detail wasn't particularly important to me. It was a routine experience. I've driven over that bridge hundreds of times. As it is with brushing our teeth, taking a shower, getting dressed, drinking our morning coffee, and commuting in the evening—because these experiences are essentially the same day-to-day, we don't pay attention to them. And because we don't pay attention to them, we don't remember them. We tend to pay attention to—and therefore remember—what we find interesting, meaningful, new, surprising, significant, emotional, and consequential. Our brains capture those details. We ignore, and therefore forget, the rest.

In 1980, my father began a new job as vice president of development at a high-tech company. Filling out forms with someone from personnel, he wrote down his phone number without hesitation, but when he got to the line prompting him for his address, he was stumped. He didn't know his street address, and he had lived there for *five years.* My father wasn't an older man with Alzheimer's. He was a thirty-nine-year-old brilliant executive. The woman in personnel refused to believe that he didn't know where he lived. My father explained that of course he did.

"You drive down Trapelo Road, then you take a left at the bottom of the hill and then the first right. My house is the third on the left." He said he had never committed the street name or number to memory, because it wasn't important.

Amused, the woman from personnel asked him, "Well, what color is your house?"

After a long pause, my dad smiled and said, "I don't know, but I can give you my phone number, and my wife can tell you."

He still defends himself. "I don't pay attention to that kind of stuff."

How could my father drive to and from his house every day for five years—that's at least 1,825 times—and not know what color it was? How could he not remember the number or the street name after that many exposures? Repetition definitely fortifies memory, but first you have to create a memory to strengthen, and without attention, that doesn't happen. Because my father never paid attention to the house color, street name, or number, this information was never consolidated into memory to begin with.

If my father's experience seems like a far-fetched example of absentmindedness, here's perhaps a more relatable example. Remember the penny I asked you to imagine earlier? Unless you're an avid penny collector—someone who regularly examines and cares about the features of pennies—you probably had a hard time recalling exactly what it looks like from memory. Let me make it easier. Look at these seven pennies.

Six are bogus. Can you recognize which penny is the real deal? You're not entirely sure, are you?

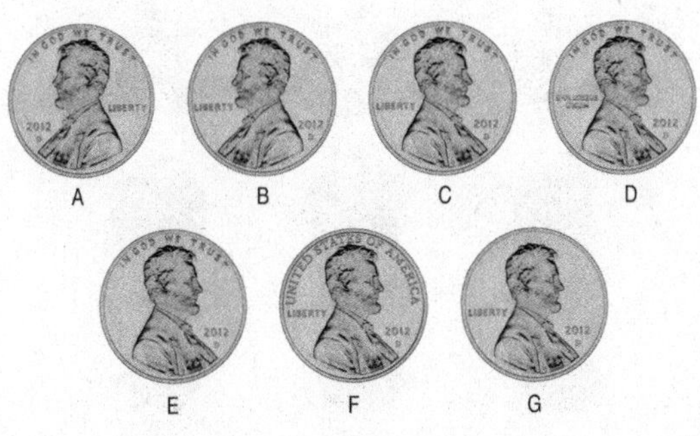

In the original 1979 penny test, less than half of the subjects identified the actual penny in a similar lineup. The real penny is C. If you're like the folks who couldn't remember where the word LIBERTY is situated or whether Lincoln's profile faces right or left, don't feel bad. These features are of no consequence to you. They don't affect the penny's value or your ability to spend it, and because the details on the front and back of a penny hold no meaning for you, you never paid attention to them. Despite thousands of exposures to pennies over decades, without your attention, you never created a memory for this information.

Here's another example likely to resonate more with younger people. The Apple logo is one of the most recognizable, ubiquitous images worldwide, and most of us see this image daily on laptops, on iPhones, and in advertisements. Whether you are younger or older, try drawing the Apple logo from memory. How confident are you that your depiction is 100 percent accurate? Now see if you can recognize which Apple is the real logo among these nine.

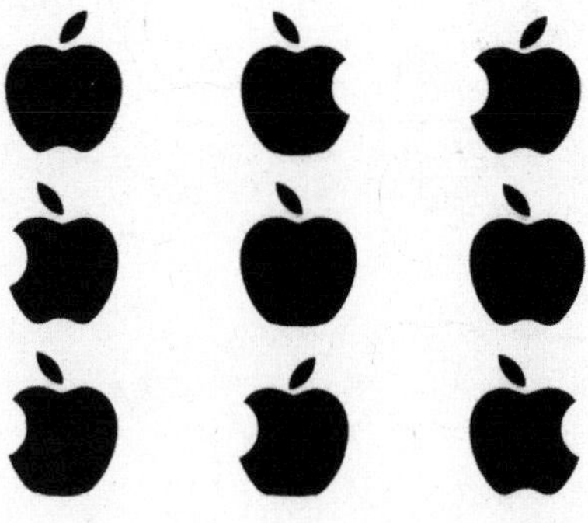

In the original test, only one out of eighty-five undergraduate students could draw the Apple logo perfectly from memory.* And as we saw with the penny test, when given several variations to choose from, less than half (47 percent) could identify the real McCoy. How did you do? If you picked any of these apples, you're wrong. All nine are fake.

What does it mean that so few people could identify this ubiquitous icon? Has Apple done a pitiful job in marketing its logo to the consumers of the world? Of course not. We all know an Apple product when we see one. But we remember the gist of the logo or the penny as a whole and don't necessarily retain the details. Repeated exposure alone simply isn't enough to guarantee that we will remember something. We need to add attention.

Now let's consider a hypothetical example that will probably feel all too familiar. You're at a party, and your friend Sarah introduces you to her husband. "Hi, I'm Bob," he says. You tell him your name and shake hands. Two minutes later, you're still chatting with him, and you realize, to your shame and horror, that you have no idea what his name is.

Or this happens: You bump into him a few days later at the grocery store. He says with a big smile, "Hi, [Your Name]!"

* Of the eighty-five students in this study, fifty-two were religious Apple users, twenty-three were Apple and PC agnostic, and ten were devout PC users. There was no difference among any of these groups in their ability to recall or recognize the Apple logo.

You recognize him. You know you met him at that party. He's Sarah's husband. But you cannot recall his name. You say, "Hey, *you*!"

Why couldn't you remember Bob's name? You clearly heard him say, "Hi, I'm Bob." Your ears weren't clogged. Your auditory cortex received the sounds of the words, and the areas of your brain that process language comprehended what was said.

But it's not enough to be exposed to the sound of Bob's name. To remember his name, you have to pay attention to it. Once the name is spoken, you'll have the sound of Bob's name available in your brain for about fifteen to thirty seconds. If you don't add the neural input of your attention, Bob's name will quickly disappear into the ether. His name will never be consolidated by your hippocampus and stored as a memory. So you didn't actually forget Bob's name. Because you didn't pay attention, you never committed his name to memory in the first place.

Paying attention requires conscious effort. Your default brain activity is not attentive. Your inattentive brain is zoned out, daydreaming, on autopilot, and full of constant background, repetitive thinking. You can't create a new memory in this state. If you want to remember something, you have to turn your brain on, wake up, become consciously aware, and pay attention.

Because we remember what we pay attention to, we might want to be mindful about what we focus on. Optimists pay attention to positive experiences, and so these events are consolidated into memory. If you're depressed, you're less likely to consolidate happy events or pleasant experiences into memory because happiness doesn't jibe with your mood. You don't even notice the sunnier moments when you're only focusing on the dark clouds. You find what you look for. If you look for magic every day, if you pay attention to the moments of joy and awe, you can then capture these moments and consolidate them into memory. Over time, your life's narrative will be populated with memories that make you smile.

We live in a constantly connected, go-go-go time plagued by distraction. Your smartphone, Facebook, Twitter, Instagram, text alerts, e-mails, incessantly racing thoughts—all of these are attention thieves and, by extension, memory thieves. Minimizing or removing things that distract you will improve your memory. Getting enough sleep, meditating, and a little caffeine (not too much and none twelve hours before bed) are powerful distraction fighters and can enhance your ability to pay attention and therefore to establish long-term memories.

People in my generation (X) regularly boast about multitasking as if it were a superpower. Likewise, millennials see no problem with watching Netflix while Snapchatting while talking to you. But there is a problem with both scenarios if you want to remember any of what you're doing and experiencing. Divided attention while your brain is trying to create a memory will significantly decrease the likelihood that it will happen. And if the information does manage to get consolidated while your attention is divided, then the memory probably won't be robust enough to be fully retrieved later. You need focused attention to lay down a memory with strength and accuracy.

So if you really want to remember what I'm saying, put down your phone. And the next time you can't find your car, pause. Before you accuse your memory of failing, before you berate it for being pathetic, before you panic and worry that you have Alzheimer's, think, *Did I pay attention to where I parked my car to begin with?*

3

In the Moment

While attention is necessary for the creation of a new memory, it isn't sufficient. Just because the beautiful sunset captured my attention on that first night of summer on the beach doesn't mean that I'll remember that sunset five years or even five minutes later. Beyond the input of your attention, the processing of information or an experience into a lasting memory begins in the here and now.

Remember Henry Molaison, the man who had both hippocampi surgically removed in an effort to eliminate his seizures? Without a hippocampus, he couldn't create any new, consciously held long-term memories. New people remained strangers forever. He couldn't retain new vocabulary, new songs, the plot of a movie, or what happened yesterday.

But he didn't lose his memory for everything. For example, he could repeat a phone number or a short list back to his doctor. Of course, a minute later, he would have completely forgotten both the phone number and that he'd ever had a conversation with his doctor about this. But he could hold ten numbers in his brain for at least a few seconds.

He could remember anything for a brief moment, a smidge longer if he constantly repeated it. He could retain information long enough to finish a coherent sentence, to comprehend what people were saying to him, and to follow directions as long as he wasn't distracted or interrupted. But how could he remember anything without a hippocampus? How could he remember anything new at all, even for a few seconds? Molaison's hippocampi were gone, but he still had his prefrontal cortex, and this is where the present moment is remembered.

Whatever is held in your consciousness right now is called your working memory. You don't retain what happened last week, last night, or even a minute ago here. Working memory only holds what you are paying attention to right now.

And then now.

This is your memory for the present moment. It's a limited and short-lived holding space in your prefrontal cortex for the sights, sounds, smells, tastes, emotions, and language of right now. It is constantly on the job, working to keep whatever you just experienced and paid attention to only long enough to use it or not.

For example, working memory carries the beginning of the sentence you are reading now long enough for you to understand the entire sentence by the time you reach the end of it. It stitches one moment to the next, giving you a contiguous understanding of what's going on. It allows you to follow a conversation, to comprehend the plotline of a movie, and to multiply twelve by fourteen in your head. You use your working memory to keep a phone number or passcode in your consciousness just long enough to enter the numbers into your phone or computer before they vanish from your mind.

You can actually feel the fleeting nature of working memory when something like the following happens. Imagine that someone rattles off a random ten-character Wi-Fi password that you need, and you have no pen in hand. You're now in a mental mad dash, rapidly repeating the first few characters in your head as you feel an invisible timer ticking down, your breath held in suspense as you scramble to enter all those letters and numbers before they evaporate. *Can you tell me that password again?*

Psychologists call working memory for what you see your *visuospatial scratchpad.* Imagine words on a sticky note hastily written in disappearing ink. Working memory for what you hear is called your *phonological loop*, the auditory version of the visual scratchpad. It's that brief echo in your head of what you just heard, the world's shortest soundtrack.

Information can't be held in working memory for long. You can hold visual information in the scratchpad and auditory information in your phonological loop for only about fifteen to thirty seconds. That's it. And then the contents are displaced by the next piece of incoming information. Life keeps happening. You keep hearing and seeing and thinking and experiencing what's going on around you and inside you. (You know you're always talking to yourself in there, right? See how you just answered me?) The next piece of data enters your working memory, and it elbows out whatever was in there before.

You can sustain the same information longer in your working memory by repeating it, either aloud or in your head. Let's say you're trying to remember that password again. Like refreshing a web page on your browser, repeating the password essentially enters the information into your present moment again, resetting the timer for another fifteen to thirty seconds. And if you repeat it enough times, the password will be consolidated via your hippocampus into a longer-lasting memory.

If Henry's doctor had said to him, "Touch your nose," he could have remembered the instruction long enough to do it successfully, especially if he had repeated the instructions to himself. He would have still been able to perceive and understand new information in the moment, thanks to working memory. But he could not have consciously recalled anything past its limited holding capacity. A minute later, that instruction would have been gone from Henry's brain. He wouldn't have been able to remember touching his nose or that his doctor had asked him to do this.

In addition to having a really short life span, working memory doesn't accommodate a lot of stuff. How much information can your working memory hold at once? The answer is as surprisingly small as it is specific. The holding capacity of working memory was first determined by George Miller in 1956, and his findings have stood the test of time. We can only remember seven plus or minus two things for fifteen to thirty seconds in working memory.

Wait, you say. Phone numbers are ten digits. Do you have an exceptional, genius-level working memory because you can accurately recall a new phone number after only hearing it once? Sorry, no.

That magical number of seven plus or minus two can be increased by chunking any information to be remembered into organized buckets or meaningful groups. We do this all the time. For example, you don't try to remember a phone number as a continuous string of ten numbers like this:

6175554062

You remember them like this:

617-555-4062

So a ten-digit phone number can fit in working memory because it's bundled as three items instead of ten—the area code plus the first three numbers plus the last four numbers. And you typically add some rhythm and melody to the sound of the phone number in your phonological loop, which helps.

Similarly, this string of numbers 12062007 will be much harder to hold in working memory than 12/06/2007 would be. When the numbers are chunked into three meaningful units like this, we easily remember them as December 6, 2007.

Here's perhaps a more compelling example. In fifteen seconds, can you remember these eighteen letters in correct order?

ALMNVYESIGIANEAOSM

What if I give you thirty seconds?

Unless you're a trained memory champion, I'm betting you still can't. What if I arrange those same letters like this:

MY NAME IS LISA GENOVA

Now can you repeat them back in order? Easy peasy. Five meaningful, bundled chunks fit easily and neatly inside working memory. But you can't stuff eighteen meaningless letters inside that same suitcase. The first few letters will have fallen out by the time you're reading the last.

So, you can fit more information in your working memory if you can chunk the items to be remembered. Conversely, you can fit and therefore remember *fewer* than the magical seven plus or minus two items if the words you're dealing with take you longer to pronounce. Your phonological loop can manage however many words you can say in about two seconds, and it can then hold these words for fifteen to thirty seconds before the soundtrack fades.

Let's say you're trying to remember a list of items using your working memory. It's going to be harder if the words on that list have more syllables. On average, people demonstrate about 90 percent recall for a list of five monosyllabic words from working memory. Performance drops to 50 percent for a list of five words that each have five syllables. Retention decreases because it takes longer to articulate a five-syllable word in your head.

For example, without rehearsing, read the following list once and see if you can repeat it back immediately from memory:

Spoon
Ball
Pen

Rug
Door
Toy

Easy, right? Did you hear the phonological loop playing the soundtrack of the words in your head? Now do the same—without rehearsing or looking back over it—with this list:

Personality
Orthopedic
Architectural
Imagination
Astrological
Excruciating

Feel the difference? Could you sense that the beginning of this list was fading to black at around *astrological*? Maybe you're thinking that the first list was much easier to remember than the second list because the items on the first list are easier to visualize, and you suspect that visualization assists with memory consolidation and retrieval. This is absolutely true for remembering information that persists beyond a few seconds, but within present-moment working memory, there's no time for that. Additional processing isn't involved. To be fair, try this list:

Nice
Sad
Help
Fun
Cool
Safe

Still easy like the first list, yes? While visual cues and associations have a profound effect on consolidation and retrieval of long-term memories, they don't come into play in working memory.

Now, without looking back, can you recall all six words that were on that easy first list? Assuming it's taken you more than thirty seconds to arrive at this paragraph from the word *spoon*, then the six words on that list are no longer held in working memory. If you remember them, it's because your hippocampus is now processing them for long-term storage.

You saw that you can easily retain the sentence MY NAME IS LISA GENOVA in working memory. What happens with longer, more complex sentences? The more syllables a word, a sentence, or a list has, the more difficult it will be to remember in your working memory. Have you ever read a long-winded sentence containing many multisyllabic words and found that you had to go back to the beginning to reread the sentence in fits and starts to comprehend it? Try reading this sentence from pages 15 to 16 of *Enlightenment Now*, by Steven Pinker:

> Of all these states, the ones that we find useful from a bird's-eye view (such as one body being hotter than the other, which translates into the average speed of the molecules in one body being higher than the average speed in the other) make up a tiny fraction of the possibilities, while all the disorderly or useless states (the ones without a temperature difference, in which the average speeds of the two bodies are the same) make up the vast majority.

Did it feel cumbersome for your brain to comprehend in one pass (or even many)? Why did it feel so difficult? Even chunked, this sentence is too long and complex to fit the entire thing within the span of working memory. By the time you reach the end of the sentence, you've forgotten the beginning. And so you have to backtrack and reread to comprehend it fully.

Let's try a shorter, simpler sentence. Below is the first sentence from *Still Alice*:

> Even then, more than a year earlier, there were neurons in her head, not far from her ears, that were being strangled to death, too quietly for her to hear them.

Your brain probably made sense of that sentence in one try because by the time you reached the end of the sentence, you could still hold and remember the words from its beginning. The words between each of the commas create six manageable chunks, and the whole sentence can be spoken in about seven seconds—well within the capacity of working memory. But then, after you've read and comprehended it, a few seconds will pass, and this sentence will slip out of your consciousness.

If you've read *Still Alice*, you probably couldn't have recalled the preceding sentence from memory. You didn't memorize the words as you read them. This isn't how we read. The sentences you read are discarded from your working memory almost immediately after you read them.

We watch movies in a similar manner. I watched *The Avengers* last night with my kids. Less than twenty-four hours later, I don't think I can recall any exact dialogue. Not one line.

But wait. If everything vanishes from working memory within a few seconds, how are you going to remember anything from this book? Why read anything? How can I remember what I ate for breakfast this morning, the new jazz number my dance teacher choreographed last week, or the talk I gave at TED in 2017? Life isn't a series of lists or phone numbers to be recalled every fifteen to thirty seconds.

So what is working memory for? It is the gateway to memory as most of us think of it. Details available in your present moment that capture your attention and have special meaning or emotion attached can be plucked from the doomed fate of working memory and sent to your hippocampus. There they are consolidated into a long-term memory, which, unlike your working memory, is thought to have limitless duration and capacity.

Right now, I'm typing these words on my computer in my kitchen. I see my hands, the computer, my Starbucks venti cup, an unanswered text alert on my iPhone, and that the time is 3:34. I hear a lawn mower, the sound of the computer keys clicking as I type, and the hum of the refrigerator. I feel hungry. This is my present moment, and this information will be held in my working memory for fifteen to thirty seconds. If nothing about this moment is, well, momentous, then that information will disappear from my working memory, my consciousness, my brain, almost instantly and forever. I won't remember it.

If, however, something about this moment is worth keeping—if I'm typing the final sentence of this book, if that text message says that Jessica Chastain wants to star in the film adaptation of one of my novels, if I write about this moment in a chapter that I'll reread and edit dozens of times (that amount of repetition should do it), then the information I perceived and found significant in this moment will shuttle from the temporary space of working memory to my hippocampus, where neurons can then link these fleeting and disparate pieces of sensory information into a single memory—the story of what happened today in my kitchen. And now, instead of forgetting everything about this moment in thirty seconds, I might remember this present moment for decades.

4

Muscle Memory

If paid attention to and meaningful enough, the present moment can be consolidated into a stable, long-lasting memory. We have three basic types of long-term memories: memory for information, memory for what happened, and memory for how to do things.

I love to ski. I learned on a pair of old Dynastars handed down from my cousin Kathleen when I was in sixth grade. I skied primarily in New Hampshire through high school, Maine while in college, and anywhere in New England into my twenties. But then I had three children and moved to Cape Cod, where the only hills are sand dunes, and the next thing I knew, I blinked and hadn't skied in over a decade.

When I finally got back in the skiing saddle, I remember standing atop the first run, staring down at the steep, icy pitch, fear ringing the bells of my sympathetic nervous system as I not-so-confidently wondered, *Do I still remember how to do this?* I took a breath, pointed my hips and tips forward, and, without thinking about how I would get there, skied to the bottom. I know I must have had a thrilled grin on my face as I thought, *Just like riding a bike, baby.*

Popular culture calls this ability to perform a previously learned skill *muscle memory.* With repetition and focused practice, complex sequences of previously unrelated physical movements can be bound together and executed as a single action instead of as a series of separate, labored steps. When the precise pattern is committed to memory, it can be performed fluidly, faster, more accurately, and without conscious thought about how to do it. So we can play "Für Elise" on the piano, drive to work, catch a baseball, walk to the kitchen, or ski down a mountain without devoting any conscious energy to how these things are done while we do them. In the words of Nike, we just do it. And while you might not remember what your spouse said five minutes ago, muscle memories are remarkably stable and can be called back into play even after sitting on the bench for decades.

But the term *muscle memory* is a misnomer, and I'm here to restore credit to its rightful owner. Your body can perform the Chicken Dance once you've learned the routine, and it might feel as if your arms and legs remember how to do the steps, but the program for this choreography doesn't live in your muscles. It's in your brain.

How to do the things you know how to do are memories activated in your brain, but this kind of memory is a bit different from memory as you're used to thinking about it. We typically consider memory to be the stuff we know (an octagon has eight sides, our phone number, the earth is round) and the stuff that happened (I tore my anterior cruciate ligament playing rugby in college, Pharrell Williams gave me a thumbs-up and a smile after one of my talks, I went to a wedding last weekend). These kinds of memories are called *declarative.* You can declare that you remember or know something. Retrieval of declarative memories involves the conscious recall of previously learned information and previously lived experience.

For example, who starred opposite Tom Hanks in the movie *You've Got Mail*? You're consciously searching for the memory in your brain, and you'll consciously know when you land on it. If this question was too easy and you instantly knew that the answer was Meg Ryan, try this one: Who starred opposite Tom Hanks in *Splash*? Or, list everyone you texted yesterday. You feel the conscious effort to find this information.

Attempts to retrieve these kinds of memories itch us where we can't quite scratch on a daily basis. Why did I come into this room? What's that guy's name? Where did I leave my phone? Recalling declarative memories can feel labored, maddening, and sometimes fruitless. We're conscious of the effort as we try to hunt the memory down, and our relationship with retrieving the stuff we know and the stuff that happened is often one of dread and hard work.

Muscle memory is different. This is your memory for motor skills and procedures, the choreography of how to do stuff. Muscle memory is unconscious, remembered below your awareness. Driving a car, riding a bicycle, eating with chopsticks, hitting a fastball, brushing your teeth, and typing are all muscle memories. Once upon a time, you didn't know how to do these things. Then, through a lot of repetition and refinement, you learned. You committed the steps to memory. And now, when you go to ride a bike, you don't have to stop and think, *Wait, let me recall how to do this first.* Similarly, U.S. gymnast Simone Biles doesn't have to think about how she's going to twist and turn her body as she's vaulting herself into the air. Once learned, the steps are retrieved instantly, effortlessly, and unconsciously. You are utterly unaware of these memories while remembering them. They become automatic, rote. You hop on the bike and go. Biles executes a Yurchenko full and sticks the landing.

So how and where are muscle memories made? Let's say you're learning how to play golf. An instructor teaches you how to align your feet and shoulders with the ball. He shows you how to set up at a distance that allows your clubface to reach the ball while you keep your arms straight. Bend your knees.

Not that much. Relax your grip. Keep your eyes on the ball. You learn how to rotate your torso and execute the backswing, the downswing, and the follow-through.

To create a highly accurate, repeatable, automated pattern of movement that in this case is hitting a golf ball, the sequence of individual physical steps must become connected—linked together into a single retrievable memory. While semantic and episodic memories are consolidated via the hippocampus, muscle memories are bound together by a part of the brain called the basal ganglia. As the sequence of physical steps is practiced, it is translated into a connected pattern of neural activity. As you continue to learn the skill, another part of the brain called the cerebellum provides additional feedback. *Stand a little more to the left. Don't bend your wrist.* Adjustments and refinements in movement are made. And you improve.

While the hippocampus is essential for forming new episodic and semantic memories, this brain structure isn't involved at all in creating muscle memories. Henry Molaison, the young man who had both hippocampi surgically removed in an effort to treat his unrelenting seizures, was never again able to lay down any new consciously held memories. But remarkably, he could still create new muscle memories. He couldn't remember what happened five minutes ago, but he could still learn how to do new things.

In psychologist Brenda Milner's most famous example, she taught Henry how to mirror-draw. He was asked to trace a star by drawing within the space between two other concentric stars drawn on a piece of paper, but he could only see these stars and his paper and pencil through their reflection in a mirror. This task isn't easy, and Henry wasn't very good at doing it at first, but he improved with continued practice and could eventually mirror-draw the star error-free. So he could learn, which demonstrated that he could create and retain a long-term muscle memory for how to mirror-draw this star. But, as with every experience since his surgery, he had no conscious memory of ever having learned how to do this. Every single time he drew that star, he claimed it was the very first time he had ever done it. His unconscious muscle memory remembered what his conscious declarative memory forgot.

So, consolidation of muscle memories requires repeated activation through lots of focused practice. Once the pattern of neural activation for a skill is consolidated, the memory for how to hit a golf ball then resides in the linked activation of neurons in your motor cortex. These are the neurons that, through connections in the spinal cord, tell all the voluntary muscles of your body what to do. Wiggling your left big toe, pointing your right index finger, leaping into the air in a grand jeté, and hitting a golf ball with a club can all be mapped to the firing of distinct neurons in your motor cortex.

As with other kinds of memory, with continued repetition your muscle memories become stronger and more efficiently retrieved. And because these connected neurons tell the body what to do, you get better at doing things with practice. Practiced skills become more stable and consistent.

Some of this improvement is due to the training of the muscles in your body. If you practice running the 110-meter hurdles over and over, the muscles involved in sprinting and leaping over those hurdles become strengthened and sculpted for performing that particular skill, and you'll improve. But your ability to run over those hurdles faster and without falling has primarily developed because you've repeatedly activated and strengthened specific neural connections in your brain. You're a better hurdler not just because your quads got bigger. I can do squats all day long, develop huge quadriceps muscles, and never make it over that first hurdle cleanly. You're better at hurdling with practice because your brain got bigger.

As you progress from novice to master, brain scan studies show that the parts of your motor cortex activated by that skill become enlarged. So, for example, the part of your motor cortex responsible for movement in your fingers becomes enlarged if you're a pianist, and it takes up even more real estate if you're a virtuoso versus a novice player. Becoming an expert in any physical skill is a result of more neural connections, more brain matter devoted to that muscle memory.

Whatever you do over and over changes your brain, then your brain changes how you move your body. There's no precise prescription for how much practice is enough to change your brain, but it generally takes much more repetition to learn a new skill than it does to learn someone's name or remember where you parked your car. In his book *Outliers,* writer Malcolm Gladwell popularized the notion that it takes ten thousand hours of practice to go from novice to expert. At first glance, this number feels absurdly high. For example, I take a one-hour dance class once a week. I'll be labored and clumsy and make a lot of missteps the first time my teacher shows us the choreography to "Uptown Funk" by Mark Ronson, featuring Bruno Mars, but after two or three more classes, I'll have practiced enough to commit the routine to memory, and I'll be able to perform it with no mistakes. So that's only four hours. What's going on here? Am I the world's best dancer? Hardly.

Claiming that it only took me four hours to master the choreography to "Uptown Funk" ignores the years of dance—and muscle memory—that predated learning that particular set of steps. I began ballet and tap when I was three, performed in a dance company in high school, and danced at Jeannette Neill Dance Studio in Boston into my thirties. So my ability to expertly perform the dance routine to "Uptown Funk" recruited muscle memories cumulatively gained over the course of my life, which could conceivably add up to ten thousand hours of dance.

While there's actually nothing magical about this number, Gladwell correctly observes that with a lot of focused training and repetition, you will get significantly better at any skill you're trying to master. But will you become a master? Not necessarily. If you practiced enough, could you kick a soccer ball as well as Abby Wambach does? Or vault like Simone Biles? Maybe. But at five feet three inches, I can practice until the cows come home, and I'll never be able to dunk a basketball like Michael Jordan. Some of us are born with brains and body types predisposed to and equipped for performing certain skills better than others are. But if you stand a chance of being good at doing anything, you need plenty of deliberate, focused practice. Repetition is the key to muscle memory mastery.

Creating a muscle memory is different from how declarative memories are made. Retrieval is different, too, and remarkably so. Once learned, muscle memories are recalled without your conscious effort. How to do things is remembered but not consciously. Much is going on in my brain when I ride a bicycle. I'm retrieving the memories, activating the connected neural circuits for how to pedal, balance, steer, and brake, but I'm not consciously involved in these processes.

Say you're learning to play Schumann's Fantasie in C Major on the piano. At first, playing will take a great deal of conscious processing, focused effort, and painstaking repetition. But once you've practiced enough—once you've integrated the procedural information into your muscle memory—the remembered sequence of notes is relegated to unconscious memory. You can play the piece without looking at the sheet music and without thinking about the pattern of individual notes. You place your fingers on the keys, and you play.

We unconsciously retrieve muscle memories all day long. Are you aware of the procedure for how to read as you're reading this chapter? No. Do you have to consciously retrieve the details of the driving lessons you had when you were sixteen every time you drive your car? No. Do you consciously break down the steps for how to swing a tennis racket as you're returning a serve? No. Do you remember learning to type as you type an e-mail? Maybe you can remember learning how to type. I was in tenth grade and sat at the back of the class, to the right of my friend Stacey. I remember the tedious drills: AAA—SSS—DDD—FFF. But I don't need to recall any of these drills to type this chapter. I've committed to memory how to type. And this kind of memory is not consciously retrieved. We can type without thinking about how to type.

It's phenomenally beneficial that our brains are designed in this way. In delegating muscle memory to subconscious neural circuitry, the brain's president, CEO, and other higher-ups are free to continue their executive functions of thinking, imagining, and decision-making while you're doing what you already know how to do. So you can walk, chew gum, *and* have a conversation. I can write this book, concentrating on what I want to communicate with you, without having to think once about the mechanics of writing or typing letters and spelling words.

We come with brains unlimited in their capacity to create muscle memories. Your brain can learn how to do pretty much anything, which is kind of mind-blowing. Just as it can learn the multiplication tables or a foreign language, your brain can learn to tango, knit, throw a perfect spiral, do a handstand, ride a unicycle, fly a plane, surf, ski, and text with your thumbs. Even if you're nowhere near Olympic level in your execution of these muscle memories, you can still learn them. All of these procedures can become automated skills performed by muscles activated by unconscious memories created through repetition. With enough training, you can alter the neural connectivity in your motor cortex so that what once seemed incomprehensibly foreign and undoable is now so easy, it's like riding a bike, baby.

5

Your Brain's Wikipedia

I live in Massachusetts.

You need a hippocampus to form new consciously retrievable memories.

I have three children.

The speed of light is approximately 186,000 miles per second.

H_2O is the chemical formula for water.

Paris is the capital of France.

I am a writer.

Worldwide, almost fifty million people have Alzheimer's.

Information that is paid attention to, salvaged from the doomed fate of working memory for its perceived significance, and consolidated by the hippocampus can become stored long-term memories. These consciously held memories store the stuff you know and the stuff that happened. The stuff you know, so-called *semantic memory*, is memory for the knowledge you've learned, the facts you know about your life and the world—the Wikipedia of your brain. And you can recall this information without remembering the details of learning it. Semantic memory is knowledge disconnected from any personal when and where. It is data unattached to any specific life experience.

Memories for what happened, for information that *is* attached to a where and when are called *episodic*. You *remember* episodic memories. "Remember when we went to Budapest." Semantic memories, on the other hand, feel more like information that you just know. "Budapest is the capital of Hungary." Episodic is personal and always about the past. Semantic memory is about information and is timeless. Just the facts, ma'am.

For example, I know that the speed of light is approximately 186,000 miles per second. I pulled that information from semantic memory. If I could recall the specific circumstances of learning that nugget of information (I can't), then that would be an episodic memory.

Similarly, you know that George Washington was the first

president of the United States, but you don't remember him being president, as you weren't alive yet. And you probably don't remember the actual experience of learning this fact, because you learned it when you were a little kid, and this episodic memory has faded over time. You've forgotten the where and when and just remember what you learned. "George Washington was the first U.S. president" is a semantic memory.

Semantic memory isn't just for presidents, state capitals, math formulas, and whatever else you learned in school. This memory also houses all your personal data. I was born on November 22. I don't remember being born, but I know that the twenty-second is my birthday. All the biographical information you fill out on registration forms—name, address, phone number, date of birth, your marital status, and so forth—is retrieved from your semantic memory.

Because every piece of data in our heads is a semantic memory, if we want to know a lot of information, we have to be really good at creating *and* retrieving semantic memories. So how do we do this? Creating a long-lasting semantic memory typically requires studying and practice, often with the intentional goal of retaining the information. Memorization requires repetition and effort. But certain kinds of repetition and effort are more effective than others.

Sometimes, life naturally gives us the repetition we need to memorize information. This is how babies and toddlers learn language. It's no coincidence that first words are often *mama, dada, baba,* and *more.* Aside from being the simplest to pronounce, these words are said by parents over and over.

The Starbucks baristas I visit daily in support of my chai habit start making my drink when they see me approaching the counter. I don't have to say a word. And it's no simple order they have memorized: venti, hot, two-pump chai tea latte, coconut milk, no water, no foam (I'm embarrassed, but yes, I'm that person). When I recently asked them how many customer drink orders they have memorized, they guessed around fifty. While each barista might have different strategies for associating certain people with certain beverages, the common denominator for creating these semantic memories is repetition. These baristas know the orders for their regular customers by heart because we show up every day, giving their brains the repetition needed to memorize what we drink.

What if you can't wait for repeated, habitual life experience to gradually carve new semantic memories into your brain? We've all had the experience of studying for a test or a presentation. What if you have to learn all twelve cranial nerves, the details of the Battle of Midway, or every line of Macbeth's "Tomorrow and tomorrow and tomorrow" soliloquy for an exam next week? Which is better for long-term retention—cramming the night before or studying the material spaced out over the seven days?

If the total number of study hours is equal, distributed

practice beats out cramming. Called the *spacing effect*, rehearsing the information to be remembered spaced out over time gives your hippocampus more time to fully consolidate what you're learning. Spacing also gives you a better opportunity to self-test, which, as you'll see shortly, dramatically strengthens the circuitry of this memory.

So if you can help it, don't pull an all-nighter before a test. You might manage a good grade by regurgitating the contents of your stuffed hippocampus in the morning, but you're highly unlikely to remember this information next week or next year. Space out what you're trying to learn. You'll remember more and forget less.

You probably already knew that repeated exposure to information helps you retain it. You repeated 8 × 3 = 24 over and over when you were in the third grade, pounding the numbers into your head until you eventually memorized it. But there are better ways than brute-force rote memorization for learning information.

As you know by now, memory involves both consolidating information into your brain and retrieving information from it. Learning and remembering. To better learn new data, not only do you want to repeatedly expose your brain to the data you want to acquire but you also want to repeatedly *retrieve* this new data from your brain.

I'm talking about quizzing yourself. So it's not just 8 × 3 = 24 over and over. It's also *What is 8 × 3?* over and over. When you test yourself and get the answer right, you're retrieving information you've managed to learn, and through the act of recalling it, you're reactivating the neural pathways of that memory, reinforcing them, making the memory stronger. If you only reread what you're trying to know, you're passively seeing and perceiving the information again and again, but you're never retrieving it. As a result, you won't see that added memory-enhancing bonus. Repeated testing beats repeated studying.

Likewise, if you're introduced to a woman named Kathy, you might repeat her name as you shake her hand. "Nice to meet you, Kathy." Now you've heard her name twice. Repeating her name is helpful, but even more helpful is quizzing yourself. If you later ponder, *What's the name of that woman I met earlier?* As long as you can come up with *Kathy* and don't draw a blank, you'll be more likely to remember her name the next time you see her.

Here's an experiment that nicely illustrates this point. Subjects were tasked with learning Swahili, a language none of the subjects had had any previous experience with. They were all given forty English-Swahili word pairs to learn.

Subjects in Group 1 were shown the word pairs, *and* they tested themselves a set number of times. Think of flash cards. You see the English word and then try to say the Swahili word before looking at the back of the card.

Subjects in Group 2 stopped studying the Swahili words once they knew these words, and they continued to read the word pairs they hadn't yet committed to memory by reading them only. These folks continued studying what they hadn't yet memorized without self-testing.

Group 3 subjects were shown the word pairs the same number of times that Group 1 saw them, but they did not self-test. And Group 4 participants, like Group 2, stopped studying the Swahili words once they knew them. But Group 4 people also tested themselves on the words that they had trouble learning rather than simply rereading those words.

One week later, all four groups were tested for recall. Groups 1 and 4 (the groups that used self-testing to learn) recalled 80 percent of the Swahili words, whereas Groups 2 and 3 (the folks who did not self-test) remembered only about 35 percent. Self-testing more than doubled recall!

What else do we need in order to remember information? Meaning matters when it comes to creating and recalling any kind of memory. I can't emphasize this enough. Here's a great example. Seasoned taxi drivers and newbie taxi driver students in Helsinki were asked to recall a list of streets. If the streets were listed in a contiguous order that could actually be driven, the veteran taxi drivers recalled 87 percent of the streets when tested. The newbies only recalled 45 percent.

These results make total sense. With their greater experience, the seasoned drivers have built up more knowledge—more semantic memories—of the streets of the city. They know their way around better than the students do.

But if the veterans and newbies were given the same list of street names in *random* order—so the first street on the list doesn't physically connect to the next street on the list, and so on—then there was no difference in recall between the seasoned drivers and the students. In this case, with the street names stripped of their meaning, the veterans' retrieval advantage, which was based on the meaningful routes between the streets, was lost.

Here's another example. Chess players were asked to look for only five seconds at a chessboard set up with twenty-six to thirty-two pieces placed in realistic game positions. They were then given an empty board and asked to reproduce what they briefly saw. How good were their memories? The chess players who were masters and grand masters could replace an average of sixteen pieces correctly on the board. Novices only got three pieces. Not surprising.

But here's where it gets interesting. If the twenty-six to thirty-two pieces were arranged on the board randomly, with no playable meaning in relation to an actual game, then the masters lost their memory advantage and remembered the piece positions just as poorly as the novices did. Instead of remembering the position of sixteen pieces, they only remembered an average of three. It was the meaning of the pieces and their positions that gave the masters their memory superpowers. They don't have better memories across the board (pun intended). They have better memories for what is meaningful to them.

Your brain isn't interested in knowing what's boring or unimportant. If you want to know more stuff, make the information meaningful to you. Attaching meaning is how mnemonics work. If you play piano, you probably memorized the notes on the treble clef line by using the mnemonic "Every good boy deserves fudge" or something similar. The notes are E, G, B, D, and F. That sweet sentence is easier to learn and retain than is just the alphabetical order of the notes on the lines and spaces, because sentences have meaning. To memorize the twelve cranial nerves, I first memorized this catchy rhyme: "On old Olympus's towering top, a Finn and German viewed some hops." And then the first letters served as cues for remembering the cranial nerves in order—olfactory, optic, oculomotor, trochlear, and so on. The sentence has meaning, and that's easier to remember than the list of nerves independent of any associated cues.

Many techniques out there go beyond simple mnemonics for enhancing your semantic memory, but the most powerful of these take advantage of at least one of your brain's two greatest talents—visual imagery and remembering where things are located in space. Your brain can very easily conjure the visual image of pretty much anything you ask it to. For example, imagine Oprah Winfrey dressed in an Easter Bunny costume, chomping on a big carrot. Got her? Of course you do. Now put her somewhere. She's sitting on your kitchen counter. See her there? Easy, right? And guess what else? What you've just done . . . is highly memorable.

But how is the image of Oprah dressed as the Easter Bunny sitting on your kitchen counter useful in any way? By itself, it's not. But if you associate this visual and spatial imagery with something you're trying to memorize, then you have an incredibly powerful neural connection and cue for recalling the information you want to remember.

Remember Akira Haraguchi, the retired engineer from Japan who memorized 111,700 digits of pi? How on earth did he do that? He and other memory athletes like him use techniques that chunk and transform enormous strings of meaningless numbers into visual images. Haraguchi translates numbers into syllables, and then those syllables become words that build elaborate and meaningful stories that he can picture . . . and remember with lots and lots of daily practice.

Memory champion Joshua Foer, author of *Moonwalking with Einstein*, used another technique for memorizing information. He first memorized a *person* performing some kind of *action* on an *object* for every two-digit number from 00 to 99. Then he could chunk any six digits into a unique person-doing-something-to-something scene. So if the number 10 is Einstein riding a donkey, and 57 is Abby Wambach kicking a soccer ball, and 99 is Jennifer Aniston eating a bagel, then the number 105799 becomes Einstein kicking a bagel. The more surprising, disgusting, bizarre, ugly, active, or even impossible the images are, the more memorable.

But you would have to do a lot of memorizing before you can actually use these techniques (and others like them) to remember the stuff you're interested in remembering. If the thought of doing this kind of mental labor sounds exhausting, I'm right there with you. I don't have the dedication or time. Unless you're motivated to become an elite memory athlete or your life's dream is to memorize 111,700 digits of pi, I suspect you don't, either. Most of us will never want or need to memorize that kind or that amount of information. But many of us would like to be better at memorizing the ten things on our to-do list, our Wi-Fi password, or the six things we need at the grocery store.

A less daunting and more practical technique for memorizing the more modest kinds of lists you actually use is called *the method of loci* or *memory palace.* The ability to remember where food is located, where to hide, and the way back home to safety was probably pretty essential for early human survival. Whether you're a kid or eighty years old, a terrible student or an astrophysicist, your brain has evolved to be able to picture and remember where things are.

With the memory palace method, you're tapping into your innate superpowers of visual and spatial imagery to associate the items to be memorized with physical locations. These locations don't need to be in a palace, but they need to be in a place you already know.

If your home is your palace, visualize six locations or pit stops as you walk into and through your home. My route goes like this: my mailbox, my front doorstep, the mudroom bench, the kitchen counter, the oven, the sink. Whatever locations along the route you choose, make sure that they're in the order you would naturally follow or that you can memorize them easily.

Let's now say I have a grocery list and no phone and no paper and pencil. With no external aids, I need to remember to buy these six items—eggs, bananas, avocados, bagels, toothpaste, and toilet paper. In my mind's eye, I place the eggs in my mailbox, the bananas on my front doorstep, the avocados on the mudroom bench, the bagels—held by Oprah—on the kitchen counter (remember, we put her there earlier), the toothpaste in the oven, and the toilet paper in the kitchen sink. When I'm at the store later today, I can walk through the mental landscape of my memory palace, visiting the locations in my mind as I imagine walking into my house. And I'll "see" the eggs inside the mailbox when I open it, the bananas on the front step, and so forth.

If I don't create an external list or use this technique, I'm likely to forget to buy the bagels. Unattached to any associations, images, or places, these free-floating grocery items won't go into my brain in a rich, deeply encoded way, and as a result, they'll be more difficult to recall. The memory palace method provides elaborative encoding, associations to visual images and locations that your evolved brain loves and can use as hooks to fish out all the groceries on your list—in order, if you want to show off. Now if only you can remember to go to the store . . .

Regular use of these tools—repetition, spaced learning, self-testing, meaning, and visual and spatial imagery—will no doubt strengthen your semantic memory. You'll be able to remember more stuff. And knowing more stuff is universally considered an enviable trait. People who know more are smart people. But there is more to remember than information. Although remembering lots of information can help you score a 1600 on your SATs and possibly even land you a spot as a contestant on *Jeopardy!*, the integration of the information you know with the life experiences you remember is what makes you wise. In addition to the stuff you know, there is the stuff that happened.

6

What Happened

- I remember sledding down the middle of Trapelo Road after the blizzard of 1978.
- I remember the moment I held my oldest daughter for the first time.
- I remember the time I saw Cold Play in concert with my friend Ashleigh.
- I remember the night of the Oscars when Matthew McConaughey said, “Julianne Moore, for *Still Alice*.”
- I remember the night I met Joe.

Episodic memory, your memory for what happened in your life, is the history of *you* remembered by you. It is memory tethered to a place and time, the where and when recollections of your life's experiences. Episodic memory is time-traveling to your past. *Remember when* . . .

Some experiences stick, lasting a lifetime, whereas others slip away by the next day, totally unmemorable. How can we have such elaborately detailed, robust, readily retrievable memories for some life events and absolutely no memory for others? What determines which experiences are remembered and which go into the ash heap? Why don't we simply remember everything that happens?

Let's start with what you *don't* remember:

- What you had for dinner five Thursdays ago
- Driving your kids to school three months ago Wednesday
- Your commute to work last Tuesday
- Every time you did the laundry in April
- The shower you took Friday morning

Can you recognize what all these forgotten life experiences have in common? They are routine. We do these things all the time. These utterly unmemorable moments are the mundane, habitual events of our daily lives. While meals, personal hygiene, errands, and commuting take up much of our waking hours, they take up very little memory over the long run. Episodic memory is not interested in the same old, same old. We don't hold on to what is ordinary, typical, or expected. These experiences don't make it past the present moment.

I'm fifty years old. I've eaten over eighteen thousand dinners in my life so far. How many of these dining experiences do I specifically remember? Very few.

Spaghetti again? Snooze. Forgotten.

So what do we remember? While our brains are terrible at remembering what is boring and familiar, they're phenomenal at remembering what is meaningful, what is emotional, and what surprises us. If you think about the dinners you do in fact remember, you'll quickly realize that they are all special in some way. Otherwise, they fade to oblivion.

For example, can you tell me what you had for dinner on Thursday, November 28, 2019? Probably not, unless I remind you that this was Thanksgiving. Now, because this was a holiday and not just any Thursday but a special Thursday, you might be able to tell me everything you had for dinner on November 28, 2019. I had two pecan rolls, ravioli (we're Italian and require pasta at every meal), turkey, and a cream puff.

You can also probably tell me who was with you. Maybe what you wore. The football teams that played that afternoon and who won, maybe even the score. The weather. You got into a political argument with your uncle. You rewatched *Home*

Alone that night. How you felt about it all. Because that day had special meaning, your memory of what happened is retrievable and rich with detail.

But then if I ask you what you had for dinner on November 30, 2019, a more recent memory and only two nights after Thanksgiving, you would probably come up blank. I have no memory of what I ate, whom I ate with, what I wore, the weather, or how I felt about it all on November 30. That day was probably a ho-hum day. We don't remember ho-hum. Unless the dinner had special significance, unless something surprising or emotional happened during the meal, or unless I revisited the experience of that day by thinking about it and talking about it regularly, it is likely to be forgotten.

Part of the reason I won't remember the experience of brushing my teeth this morning has to do with habituation—we learn to ignore what is familiar and of no consequence. And we can't remember what we ignore. Remembering requires that we give the thing to be remembered our attention.

For example, let's say your husband pulls into the driveway every evening at six o'clock in his silver Toyota Camry. He does this five nights a week, week after week. You see him pull into the driveway through the kitchen window every evening at six. But you probably have no distinct memory of any particular homecoming, because they're all much the same.

Now let's imagine that he pulls into the driveway tonight at five o'clock in a red Ferrari, dressed in drag, and George Clooney is in the passenger seat. Whoa! That's never happened before! Everything about this event is astonishing. The surprise factor alone is enough to kick this particular evening into memorable-for-life, but you'll also probably tell everyone you know, relaying the story over and over. *OMG, he pulled into the driveway, and you won't believe it!* And with every retelling, you are reactivating the memory, reinforcing the neural pathways that encode the details of what you experienced, making the memory stronger.

But if your husband then continues to come home every night at five in the red Ferrari, dressed in drag with his pal George Clooney, well, even George gets to be old news (I know, hard to imagine). You'll continue to remember that first time, but you won't remember the details of the 10th, 42nd, or 112th, because you've habituated to this occurrence. It has become spaghetti dinner, morning coffee, brushing your teeth. The usual. No big deal. And no big deal is readily forgotten.

Life events infused with emotion are what we tend to remember long term—triumphs, failures, falling in love, humiliations, weddings, divorces, births, deaths. Many studies have shown that episodic memories for emotional experiences are better remembered than are neutral experiences. In general, the more emotional the event, the more vividly and elaborately detailed the memory.

Emotion and surprise activate a part of your brain called the amygdala, which, when stimulated, sends powerful signals to your hippocampus that basically communicate this: *Hey, what's going on right now is super important. You're going to want to remember this. Consolidate it!* And so your brain then captures and binds together the contextual details surrounding what you experienced—where you were, who you were with, when this happened, how you felt about it, and so on. Emotion and surprise act like a big brass marching band parading through your brain, waking up your neural circuitry to what is going on. Routine events are never emotional or surprising.

And because experiences that elicit an emotional reaction in you most likely also matter to you, you tend to revisit them. You reminisce about and retell these emotionally driven, meaningful stories, making those memories stronger.

If you experience something highly unexpected and exceptionally emotional, you might create what is known as a *flashbulb memory*. Where were you . . .

- When John F. Kennedy was killed?
- When the space shuttle *Challenger* blew up?
- When the O. J. Simpson verdict was delivered?
- When Princess Diana died?

- On September 11, 2001?
- When Trump was elected president?

Flashbulb memories aren't photographic as the name suggests, but they do contain a lot of vivid detail for episodic information—where you were, who you were with, the date, what you were wearing, what you and others said, the weather, how you felt—much more so than you remember for the day before that event or even what happened last week. For example, I can remember too many moments in painful detail from the morning of September 11, 2001, but I can't tell you anything about the morning before or the morning after.

Flashbulbs are episodic memories for experiences that were shocking and highly significant to you and evoked *big* emotions—fear, rage, grief, joy, love. These stunningly unexpected, personally important, and emotionally charged experiences become memories that feel resistant to fading and can be readily recalled years later.

Flashbulb memories don't have to be for public events. They can be personal—a car accident or the death of a parent. And they don't have to be negative or catastrophic—the day your spouse proposed or, if you're from Boston, when the Red Sox won the 2004 World Series.

But if you do have a flashbulb memory for a public event, it's because you feel a personal connection to it. Both the

O. J. Simpson trial verdict and the death of Lady Diana may've been shocking to you, but if you remember these events in Technicolor detail all these years later, then they also must feel personal to you. You had been glued to the TV for weeks, watching the O. J. Simpson trial, and you felt invested in the verdict. You watched Lady Diana marry Prince Charles all those years ago and adored her ever since from across the pond.

When I hear about a bombing in England on the news, if I remember it later, I might say to a friend, "Did you hear about the bombing in England?" I'm recalling and sharing facts, but because I live far away and can't feel the emotional impact of every global outrage, my memory of learning this news probably won't stand the test of time.

But I do have a flashbulb memory of the Boston Marathon bombing. Because Boston is my hometown and I've stood at the marathon finish line many times, I remember in vivid detail where I was, who I was with, and how I felt on that Monday in April 2013. The bombing was shocking. It evoked fear and grief, and it felt personal. I suspect that distance runners from all over the world with no connection to Boston have a flashbulb memory for this event as well. But if you're from Kansas or Argentina and if you're not a distance runner, you might know that there was a bombing one year at the Boston Marathon (a semantic memory), but you probably don't remember what was happening in your life on that day when you heard the news.

Strung together, your most meaningful episodic memories create your life story and are collectively called your *autobiographical memory.* This is your highlights reel—your first kiss, the day you scored the winning goal to clinch the championship, the day you graduated from college, your wedding day, the day you moved into your first house, the time you got that big promotion, the births of your children. The meaningful moments you keep within the chapters of your autobiographical memory aren't necessarily all tales of rainbows and unicorns. What you remember depends on the kind of life story you're creating. We tend to save the memories that feed our identity and outlook.

My friend Pat has the most positive attitude of anyone I know. I would bet that Pat's autobiographical memory is populated with laughs, appreciation, and awe. My great aunt Aggie, on the other hand, was a chronic complainer. Her life story—the meaningful memories she retained of what happened in her life—was a tale of woe (as a young child, I actually thought her name was Aunt Agony). Similarly, if you believe you're smart, you're more likely to remember the details of the times when you did something intelligent and you're more likely to forget the times you made dumb mistakes. And by continuing to recall and reminisce about the stories that illustrate how brilliant you are, you reinforce the stability of those memories and who you believe yourself to be.

Aside from the emotionally neutral, utterly unremarkable

details of our day-to-day routines and whatever is tossed aside because it doesn't jibe with the story of who we are, what else don't we remember? In terms of what happened, we remember almost nothing before the age of three and very little before the age of six. Our earliest episodic memories are the briefest short stories, sensory snapshots that are totally disconnected from the cohesive narrative starring you as the protagonist in your life. The average age for a first episodic memory that you can remember as an adult is three. Memories remembered younger than three are exceptions and usually involve the birth of a sibling, the death or serious illness of a parent, moving to a new home, an event that was highly unexpected, or a semantic memory based on stories you've been repeatedly told about yourself by others.

The thick fog of childhood amnesia lifts at about the age of six or seven. Now what is remembered gets attached to the story of you. Your memories from age seven feel more like watching the earliest episodes of Season 1 in the Netflix series of your life's memories, whereas revisiting a memory from age four might feel more like seeing a moment from an episode midseason of some other show.

Why do we retain so few memories for what happened when we were young? The development of language in our brains corresponds with our ability to consolidate, store, and retrieve episodic memories. We need the anatomical structures and circuitry of language to tell the story of what happened, to organize the details of our experiences into a coherent narrative that can then be revisited and shared later. So as adults, we only have access to memories of what happened when we owned the language skills to describe them.

Aside from flashbulbs, what autobiographical memories do we remember best? We can still remember what happened from the past couple of years pretty well, thanks to what is called the *recency effect.* We don't have to brush away too many cobwebs or dig too far into the attic to find these recently created memories, and so they're easy to grab.

But most of life's episodic memories are likely to be clustered between the ages of fifteen and thirty. Called the *reminiscence bump,* these episodes are what we remember most in life. Why is this? We don't really know, but most scientists think it's because so many meaningful firsts are packed into those years—kiss, love, car, college, sex, job, house, marriage, child. During these years, we begin to fill our life's narrative with purpose and meaning. And again, our brains remember what is meaningful.

So we need emotion, surprise, or meaning to create and keep our episodic memories. But a few people in this world require none of these elements to remember what happened. People with highly superior autobiographical memory (HSAM) can recall the details of what happened from almost every day of their lives from late childhood on. It doesn't matter whether it was September 11, 2001, or an ordinary Monday in 1986. These folks with HSAM (fewer than one hundred people in the world have been identified) remember what happened every day, no matter whether that day was extraordinary or mundane. Basically, without shock, emotion, or meaning, every day for someone with HSAM is remembered like a flashbulb memory or a first kiss.

If you give someone with HSAM a date, as long as that date falls within the person's lifetime, he or she can tell you within seconds the day of the week, the weather that day, what the person did and with whom, what happened to him or her and in the world, and how he or she felt about it all. This seemingly magical feat isn't accomplished through calendar counting, mnemonics, or practicing some special trick. And these people aren't autistic savants who have superior memories for facts and information. People with HSAM have normal memories for faces, phone numbers, tasks like remembering to call the plumber, and where they put their keys. But when it comes to remembering what happened, HSAM folks have not-yet-explainable superpowers.

For example, consider these four dates:

- July 20, 1977
- October 3, 1988
- June 15, 1992
- September 14, 2018

Can you answer each of these questions for those four dates?

- What was the day of the week?
- Can you name a verifiable news event that happened on that date or anything that happened one month before or after that date?
- What happened in your life on that date?

If you're like me, you can't come up with much. I was a freshman in college on October 3, 1988, but I have no specific memory from that date, no idea of what day of the week it was, or any memory of what was happening in the world. I'm similarly vague on the other dates. I know where I was living and what I was generally doing at the time, but I can't recall any actual memories from those specific dates.

When given this quiz, 97 percent of people with HSAM got the day of the week correct, 87 percent produced a verifiable event, and 71 percent recalled an episodic memory. Compare these results with those from us Muggles—14 percent named the correct day of the week (since the odds of being right by guessing is one in seven, this percentage is due to chance), 1.5 percent remembered a verifiable event, 8.5 percent recalled an episodic event. Pitiful.

How do people with HSAM effortlessly and accurately

retrieve the details and day of the week for almost any date in their lifetime (typically after the age of ten)?

"It's easy for me to remember every day of 1988," says Marilu Henner, TV, movie, and Broadway actor most known for her role as Elaine O'Connor Nardo in the sitcom *Taxi* and one of the few people on this planet with HSAM. "It's like asking me an address or a phone number."

When I asked her if she could remember anything from these dates, her answers came instantly.

"July 20, 1977. That was a Wednesday. I was shooting *Bloodbrothers* with Richard Gere. I'd moved to LA the month before. That weekend, I went to San Francisco with a boyfriend and Johnny Travolta."

For each date, she located the day of the week first and within seconds. Then the events of that day and the surrounding days would begin to line up and reveal themselves.

"June 15, 1992. That was a Monday. Oh my God, that was right after the LA riots. The whole city was still in lockdown. I was working on postproduction of a dance aerobics video. I was in editing all day."

September 14, 2018, was a plant, and the second this date left my lips, Marilu said, "That's when you came to see *Gettin' the Band Back Together*. It was the final weekend." And that was, in fact, the day Marilu and I had met in person for the first time, on stage, just after she performed in that wonderful musical in New York City.

Scientists have located nine brain regions that appear enlarged in people who have HSAM. But we still don't know if these bigger brain areas endow these folks with such remarkable episodic memories or if having HSAM causes the areas to become enlarged. This causal chicken-and-egg question aside, we do know that the episodic memories of HSAM people seem to be organized in their brains by category and then anchored by a date.

"It's a timeline that I feel," Marilu told me. "I don't see it. I feel it. I can go there. It lines up left to right but not visual. It works in chunks."

Marilu can remember the details of every time she has heard *Hey Jude* by the Beatles or eaten at Tom's Diner. Every calendar date is linked to the day of the week, what she ate for lunch, and which shoes she wore, all readily retrievable. She scores in the 99th percentile for remembering what happened last year—all 365 days. Emotional, meaningful, or surprising experiences aren't any easier to recall for her than are the totally mundane. They're all the same, all memorable. Most people only remember eight to ten events for any given year. This paucity of episodic memory is as unfathomable to Marilu as her abundance of episodic memory is to the rest of us.

While Marilu holds her HSAM as a prized superpower, others with HSAM feel cursed. They readily remember in excruciatingly vivid detail the very worst, most painful days of their lives—the breakups, the deaths, every mistake and regret, every loss and humiliation. For these folks, this memory superpower feels more like a Greek tragedy. They have been granted the ultimate wish of being able to remember everything that happens, and they are plagued with misery.

While Marilu can also recall every painful life moment, she doesn't dwell on those times. She chooses to learn from life's missteps and, like my friend Pat, to focus on the positive. Whether you have HSAM or not, the episodic memories you choose to spend time with is largely up to you.

Since most of us are not endowed with HSAM, how can we get better at retaining our episodic memories, both the meaningful (how you celebrated your wedding anniversary last year) and the mundane (whether you took your allergy pill this morning)? Is there anything we can do to help us remember more than eight to ten episodic memories from this year?

GET OUT OF YOUR ROUTINE. Vacation to a new city, rearrange the furniture, celebrate a half birthday, eat at a new restaurant, rent your dream car for a weekend. Ho-hum, vanilla-again days are the kiss of death to remembering what happened.

GET OFF YOUR DEVICES, AND LOOK UP. You can't remember what you don't notice, and you won't see what's happening around you if your eyes are glued to your phone. Your best friend from kindergarten might have been standing in the

Starbucks line right in front of you yesterday, but you totally missed that memorable reunion over iced lattes because you spent the entire time browsing Facebook. The average American adult today spends almost twelve hours a day in front of some kind of screen. If you're getting eight hours of sleep a night, that means you're conscious for nonscreen experience for only four hours a day. If you want to have three-dimensional, richly detailed memories of what's happening in your life, you have to get out there and live in the three-dimensional world.

FEEL IT. Emotional experiences are better remembered than neutral ones. If you want a stronger memory for the stuff that happens, get in touch with your feelings.

REHASH IT. Repetition makes your memories stronger. Reflecting over what happened, gabbing about it with your girlfriends on the phone, and regularly reminiscing about it will help you retain those memories.

KEEP A JOURNAL. Not only does jotting down even one of today's experiences in a diary increase the likelihood that you'll remember the experience in the future, but also the information you record can serve as cues for triggering recollection of whatever else happened today. Psychologist Willem Wagenaar kept a daily diary for over six years, recording 2,402 episodic events. Merely taking the time to write these daily entries was a powerful way to rehearse these episodic memories. But beyond writing each entry, he never reread what he wrote, so there weren't any additional opportunities for rehearsal. When a colleague later tested his memory, the researcher found that if he was given enough cues (he often required more than one), Wagenaar could recall 80 percent of his daily events from the past six years. Keeping a diary works!

USE SOCIAL MEDIA. I know, I know. I just told you to get off your devices. And there's definitely plenty of dark side when it comes to social media, but it can also be used as a force for good, or at least for reinforcing your episodic memories. Browsing through your Instagram or social media profiles can be a lovely stroll down memory lane, each photo and corresponding caption serving as a powerful cue, triggering recall for what happened. And the chronology of your memories is nicely preserved there, with your most recently captured experiences displayed at the top of your page, assisting your brain in figuring out when things happened. And if you're not on social media, looking through a photo album or the photos saved on your smartphone will work, too.

LIFE-LOG. Your brain isn't a video camera, and your memory isn't a recording of everything that was perceived by you. But more and more, developing technology can serve as an extension of your brain and memory, turning this sci-fi notion of life-logging into reality. Wearable cameras, audio recorders, and various apps can collect digital data from your daily activities through images, video, and sound that can later be reviewed, reexperienced, and, well, remembered. For example, small cameras typically worn around the neck can take photos and tag your location every thirty seconds, all day long, creating a digital autobiographical record of your day. Reviewing those images strengthens your memory for what happened that day and can serve as cues for memory retrieval.

Now that you understand a bit about episodic memory—how emotion, surprise, meaning, reflection, and reminiscing all play a role in your ability to remember what happened in your life—let me leave you with this. Whether it's the day that Princess Diana died, your first kiss, the night you saw Cold Play in concert, or the first time your husband came home in a red Ferrari with George Clooney, your memories for what happened . . . are wrong.

PART II

Why We Forget

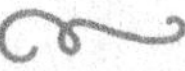

7

Your Memories (For What Happened) Are Wrong

Your episodic memories are chock-full of distortions, additions, omissions, elaborations, confabulations, and other errors. Basically, your memories for what happened are wrong. Wait a second. I've spent a lot of time in this book so far demonstrating that our brains are "pretty phenomenal" at remembering anything that is emotional, surprising, meaningful, and repeated. But now I'm telling you that your memories for what happened are wrong. Both statements are true.

Stay with me here. Understanding how and why our episodic memories are fallible can be strangely comforting. For every step in memory processing—encoding, consolidation, storage, and retrieval—your memory for what happened is vulnerable to editing and inaccuracies. To begin with, we can only introduce into the memory creation process what we notice and pay attention to in the first place. Since we can't notice everything in every moment that unfolds before us, we only encode and later remember certain slices of what happened. These slices will contain only the details that were seduced by our biases and captured our interest. So my memory for what happened last Christmas morning will be different from what my son remembers, and neither his memory nor mine will contain the full picture—the whole truth, so to speak. From the get-go, our episodic memories are incomplete.

You might then think that whatever details you noticed and captured into a memory would at least be accurate, albeit incomplete. Not at all. Think of your episodic memories as wide-eyed preschoolers who fully believe in every singing princess and giant bipedal mouse they see at Disney World. They are gullible and eager to collaborate. Nascent memories are highly susceptible to influence and creative editing, especially during the period—hours, days, and longer—when these memories are being consolidated, before they're committed to long-term memory.

In the process of consolidating an episodic memory, your brain is like a sticky-fingered, madcap chef. While it stirs together the ingredients of what you noticed for any particular memory, the recipe can change, often dramatically, with additions and subtractions supplied by imagination, opinion, or assumptions. The recipe can also be warped by a dream, something you read or heard, a movie, a photograph, an association, your emotional state, someone else's memory, or even mere suggestion.

Once stored, memories for what happened still aren't safe from alteration. Left alone for too long, memories can decay with the passage of time. The physical neural connections can literally retract and disappear, erasing part or all of your memory of what happened.

And every time we retrieve a stored memory for what happened, it's highly likely that we change the memory. As described earlier, when we retrieve a memory of something that happened, we are reconstructing the story, not playing the videotape. Memory isn't a courtroom stenographer, reading back exactly what was said. When we recall what happened, we typically fetch only some of the details we stored. We omit bits, reinterpret parts, and distort others in light of new information, context, and perspective that are available now but weren't back then. We frequently invent new information, often inaccurate, to fill in gaps in our memories so that the narrative feels more complete or pleasing. What we remember about the past is also influenced by how we feel in the present. Our opinions and emotional state today color what we remember from what happened last year. And so, in revisiting episodic memories, we often reshape them.

And then something interesting happens. We reconsolidate and restore this changed, 2.0 version of the memory and *not* the original. Reconsolidating an episodic memory is like hitting SAVE in Microsoft Word. Any edits we've made are saved to the neural circuits of that memory. The earlier version of the memory that we just retrieved is now gone. Every time we recall an episodic memory, we overwrite it, and this new, updated edition is the version we'll retrieve the next time we visit that memory.

As you might imagine, after several recalls of any given episodic memory, it has the potential to deviate quite a bit from the original. Your memory for what happened versus what actually happened can be much like the telephone game, where the original sentence becomes contaminated over several whispered relays. Just as *Red roses have thorny stems* eventually becomes *Rat horses have four neat drums* in the telephone game, the memories you share over and over with friends and family are not accurate records of what actually happened.

So how inaccurate are our episodic memories? Let me count the ways. First, through leading questions, our brains can be duped into believing they remember something we never even experienced in the first place. In several studies, researchers offered fictitious information to their subjects to see if memories could be falsely created or contaminated. The investigators told these unsuspecting folks totally fake stories about an autobiographical event, claiming to have learned these stories from parents and family.

Remember the time you went for a ride in a hot-air balloon? Remember when you got lost in a mall when you were six? Remember when you spilled red punch on the bride's dress at your cousin's wedding? Researchers asked subjects similar questions about events that never truly happened and then produced photoshopped pictures and additional details, everything completely made up. How did these subjects respond to these fictional accounts? About 25 to 50 percent of people in these studies insisted that they remembered details about these experiences that never happened!

I remember riding in that balloon. It was red. I was with my mom and little brother. When presented with leading questions, our episodic memories become those preschoolers at Disney—ready and willing to believe anything.

In another study, researchers asked subjects to share any memories they had of the video of the hijacked plane that crashed in Pennsylvania on September 11, 2001. People were interviewed and then given a questionnaire to test what they remembered. Thirteen percent offered detailed memories of the video during the interview, and 33 percent reported specific memories in the questionnaire. But 100 percent of these memories were false. We have footage of the planes that crashed in

New York City and Washington, D.C., on 9/11, but there is no video of the crash in the field in Pennsylvania. These folks believed they remembered details from a video that doesn't exist.

Because an episodic memory becomes vulnerable to outside influences every time we retrieve it, false information can also worm its way in every time we recall something, deforming the memory of what we experienced. The most common and effective smuggler of misinformation into our episodic memories is language: the words we, and others, use. In one of my favorite classic studies on this subject, two researchers showed people a video of a car accident, ensuring that all of these folks would have the same original memory of what they saw.

Later, the subjects were asked one of the following questions:

- How fast would you say the cars were going when they smashed into each other?
- How fast would you say the cars were going when they collided into each other?
- How fast would you say the cars were going when they bumped into each other?
- How fast would you say the cars were going when they hit each other?
- How fast would you say the cars were going when they contacted each other?

Memory for the speed of the cars in the video of the crash was significantly influenced by the verb used—the mere substitution of a single word. Subjects who were presented with the word *smashed* remembered the cars going ten miles per hour faster than did subjects who heard the word *contacted.* People reconstructed their memory of what happened to match the intensity of the verb offered, incorporating this adjustment into their memory during recall.

In a similar study, three groups of subjects were shown a video of a crash involving multiple cars.

- The first group was asked, "How fast were the cars going when they smashed into one another?"
- The second group was asked, "How fast were the cars going when they hit one another?"
- The third group wasn't asked any questions about the speed of the cars.

A week later, they were all asked this same question:

- "Did you see any broken glass in the video?"

Thirty-two percent remembered broken glass if they had previously been asked, "How fast were the cars going when they smashed into one another?" If they had been asked, "How fast were the cars going when they hit one another?"

only 14 percent remembered broken glass, the same as the group not asked any question about speed. As you might guess by now, there was no broken glass in the video. So everyone who remembered broken glass remembered seeing something that they never actually saw.

Since it's quite easy to manipulate episodic memory with language and misleading questions, we wouldn't want to rely on it to determine important matters such as courtroom verdicts and prison sentencing, right? Almost half of Americans believe that the testimony—and therefore the memory—of a single eyewitness alone is enough to convict a defendant. As of September 2019, there have been 365 convicted, innocent people exonerated through DNA testing in the United States. Of those, approximately 75 percent had been found guilty on the basis of eyewitness testimony. Thus, all these eyewitness memories were wrong.

In a study published in 2008, researchers showed subjects a video of a fake crime in a supermarket. The "thief" stole a bottle of liquor. There were two bystanders in the video. One walked down the liquor aisle; the other was standing in the produce section. Subjects were later shown a lineup of men, none of whom was the thief. Again, the thief was *not* in the lineup. Of the subjects tested, 23 percent picked out the innocent bystander who had walked down the liquor aisle, and 29 percent picked out the guy who had been standing in the produce section. So over half chose the wrong guy—based on their memory of what happened.

I'm not saying that the episodic memories of all eyewitnesses are wrong. But certainly, some of these memories are. In another study, people watched a thirty-second video of a bank robbery. Twenty minutes later, half of the subjects were given five minutes to write down what they saw. The other half were kept busy for an equivalent amount of time on an unrelated task. Then, everyone was asked to pick out the bank robber from a lineup. Among the nonwriters, 61 percent picked out the robber, but only 27 percent of the writers did. Note that not even a half hour later, at best only about two-thirds of people who witnessed the bank robbery could remember correctly what the robber looked like. And writing about what they had seen dramatically compromised their ability to accurately remember what they had witnessed only a few minutes earlier.

Writing something down allows you to rehearse and therefore strengthen the memory for the details you choose to write about, but this action can also unwittingly prevent you from rehearsing, and therefore later remembering, any details you didn't include. Putting any sensory experience into words distorts and narrows the original memory of the experience. As a writer, I find this phenomenon more than a little disheartening.

Likewise, even talking about your memory of what happened slices the memory thinner. The spoken story of what happened is first narrowed by language's limited capacity to describe the imagery, sounds, smells, feelings, and other impressions of any experience. And we cherry-pick only certain details when we describe what occurred.

After we talk about something that happened, this slimmer version of the memory is saved, and so we lose the fuller, original memory. Then, the next time we talk about this memory, maybe we leave out a detail. You don't mention that it had been raining. When we go to retell what happened a third time, the rain is gone from the memory. So as soon as an episodic memory leaves my lips, it contains less information than the original memory had.

But then an episodic memory can also expand with information I creatively supply or borrow from other sources. I might add a nugget of information, some background or interpretation, an embellishment that makes the story a bit better, or some new information I learned from a friend. That new detail now becomes embedded in the memory for that event in my brain.

Let's say you're sharing a story from your childhood about the time you and your brother ambushed the florist at your front door with plastic discs shot from a toy gun (we're so sorry!), and your brother says, "Yeah, and she wouldn't stop ringing the doorbell." You don't remember that, but you believe him. The next time you recall this memory, you've got that florist incessantly ringing the bell. This is now how *you* remember this event.

Or say there was a fire in your office building two days ago and everyone was evacuated. You remember exiting the building calmly, standing in the parking lot for about an hour, feeling mildly inconvenienced, not knowing if the evacuation was a drill or was due to an actual fire. Yesterday, when your coworker told the story, he shared that someone had been smoking a turkey in the office cafeteria and the smoker had caught fire. The entire kitchen was up in flames and smoke was everywhere. Your office is just down the hall from the kitchen. You could have been killed!

Today when you share your memory of the fire, you describe how you could barely see your way to the stairwell through the smoke. This common kind of memory error is called a *confabulation.* Information provided by your coworker wriggled its way into your episodic memory. You're not consciously lying. Again, episodic memory is a wide-eyed preschooler, and preschoolers believe in Santa. Your memory of this office fire now believes that the air was thick with smoke as you tried to reach the stairwell.

As you can see, with every recall, our memories for what happened can shrink, expand, and morph in all kinds of interesting and often inaccurate ways, deviating significantly from the original unspoken memory first created in our brains.

Ironically, if you jot down what happened today, you'll probably limit what you remember about today to the details you've chosen to record. Whatever you talk about will be reinforced, but that memory will deform as you continue to gab. But memories not repeated or shared at all are likely headed for the ash heap. When it comes to our memories for what happened, imperfect is the best our brains can do.

But what about flashbulb memories, those confident, vividly colored memories for emotionally charged or surprising events? Are they sturdier than your run-of-the-mill episodic memory, or are they similarly prone to editing and misinformation? Flashbulbs definitely feel much more intensely remembered than do ordinary episodic memories, even years later, and this feeds our strong belief in their durability and accuracy. They must be much more faithful to the truth than regular episodic memories are, because they're so richly detailed, right? But this confidence is mistakenly placed. Flashbulb memories are just as incomplete, distorted, and dead wrong as ordinary episodic memories are.

Consider this: On Tuesday, January 28, 1986, at 11:39 A.M., the space shuttle *Challenger* lifted off into the clear blue Florida sky carrying seven astronauts, including Christa McAuliffe, who was also the first teacher to go to space. Seventy-three seconds into the flight, just after the crew received the OK from mission control to go to full throttle, the main fuel tank exploded. Ghostly white plumes snaked through the sky as the entire spacecraft disintegrated and the world watched. There were no survivors.

Thirty-five years later, here is my flashbulb memory of the *Challenger* explosion. It was lunchtime, and I was in my high school cafeteria. I was carrying a plate of french fries and ketchup on my tray when I saw the explosion. A TV had been set up in the cafeteria so that students and teachers could watch this historic event. I remember the silence and the horror.

Not bad for a Tuesday in January thirty-five years ago, especially since I couldn't tell you a single detail from the day before or after. But is any of this information from my memory accurate?

As a sophomore in high school, I could very easily have had a lunch period at 11:40 A.M. So this part of my account is probably correct, but I know enough about episodic memory not to insist on it. Because I didn't keep a diary back then and there's no other record of what I witnessed that morning, I have no way to be certain that there was actually a TV in my high school cafeteria, that I had been eating french fries (1986 was definitely before I learned about healthy eating habits!), or that I was even in the cafeteria when the *Challenger* exploded. The details of this flashbulb memory are just as likely to be true, false, or misshapen. In fact, if I had to place money on it, I would bet that at least one totally false detail has infiltrated this flashbulb memory.

Here's why. I didn't record what I witnessed on that tragic

day, but psychologists Ulric Neisser and Nicole Harsch did. Twenty-four hours after the shuttle exploded, they asked a number of Psychology 101 students at Emory College a series of questions:

- Where were you?
- What were you doing?
- Who was with you?
- How did you feel?
- What time of day was it?

They also asked the students to rate their confidence in the accuracy of each answer, from 1 (just guessing) to 5 (certain).

Then, in the fall of 1988, two and a half years later, they gave these same students the same questions and checked their answers—their episodic memories—against their original memories. How reliable were their episodic memories? No one scored 100 percent, meaning that after two and a half years, no one gave answers that completely matched their answers at twenty-four hours. Twenty-five percent had a score of zero. Every answer these folks gave was different from what they had reported immediately after the explosion. Their memories of this event only two and a half years later were totally inaccurate. Half of the students could correctly remember their answers to only one of the questions.

As an added twist, the experimenters asked the students if they had ever answered these questions before. Only 25 percent said that they had, and 75 percent were certain that they had never seen this questionnaire before.

So there were *a lot* of errors in the memories of these young adults only a couple of years later. How accurate do you think my memory of this explosion is, with thirty-five years under its belt? I remember being in the high school cafeteria, eating french fries, and watching the explosion on TV with my classmates. But maybe I was home sick from school that day, eating chicken noodle soup alone in the kitchen at 11:40, and I watched the explosion on the news with my brother and parents that night. Even more than three decades later, I feel highly confident of the accuracy of my flashbulb memory of the explosion. But does my high level of confidence mean that my memory is accurate?

It doesn't. You can be 100 percent confident in your vivid memory and still be 100 percent wrong. If we go back to the Emory students, regardless of how they scored for accuracy, they had a high degree of confidence in what they reported remembering—even where they were shown to be dead wrong.

In the spring of 1989, these same students were presented with both sets of their answers to the questionnaire. When they were confronted with the many discrepancies between their newer memory of the explosion and their original account, they believed in the accuracy of their most recently recalled memory, the version that is wrong. Neisser and Harsch incorrectly assumed that the details of the original—in the students' own handwriting, no less—would serve as a powerful cue for the students, triggering the accurate recall of what they had actually witnessed on January 28, 1986. But this didn't happen. These folks all stuck with their more recent stories and scratched their heads over the mismatch, dumbstruck over their own original account. "I still think of it as the other way around" said one. Their memories were permanently changed. And wrong.

But knowing what we now know about episodic memory, this belief in the accuracy of the revised memory makes perfect sense. Every time we pull an episodic memory from the cortical shelf, it becomes vulnerable to change, and before it's reshelved, we overwrite the version we just retrieved with this new edition containing any updates we've made. So, assuming everyone talked or thought about the space shuttle explosion at least once after filling out that original questionnaire, then the original account of the explosion has been long erased, replaced with newer versions of the memory, updates that can unwittingly drift further and further away from what actually happened.

Let's say you and a friend from high school are reminiscing about the time you drove to see Jimmy Buffett in concert twenty years ago. Let's also say that you hadn't thought about that memory since going to the concert. In sharing the memory, your friend offers a detail that triggers part of that experience that you had forgotten about.

She says, "Remember, Jen came with us."

You say, "Oh my God, that's right! I totally forgot she was there, but now I remember. She was in the back seat!"

That detail is still stored in your brain but the neural associations connecting "Jen" to the rest of this memory were weaker and not readily activated on your own without an additional cue. Of course, as you should know by now, both of you could be wrong. Maybe Jen went with you to the Rolling Stones concert, not the Jimmy Buffett concert. Or she was in the front seat, not the back. Nevertheless, what you can recall depends a great deal on the retrieval cues available to you.

Let's say Jen did, in fact, ride with you to this concert. Now let's say that instead of not thinking about that memory for two decades, you reminisced about this concert many times over the past twenty years, but each time, you failed to include Jen in the memory you retrieved. Remember, you strengthen and reconsolidate the newest version with every recall. Because you forgot to include Jen in any of these updates, you might have lost this detail permanently. "Jen" might no longer be even weakly associated with this memory. In this case, you are likely not to believe your friend's memory of the event.

"No, Jen wasn't in the back seat!" you would say. "I'm sorry, I don't remember her being there at all." You'll stick to the story of the memory as you remember it, even in the face of strong evidence to the contrary, much like the Emory students who wouldn't believe their own handwritten accounts of the *Challenger* explosion from a couple of years earlier.

In summary, your memory for what happened might be right, completely wrong, or somewhere in between. So the next time your spouse insists they remember what happened and your spouse's story doesn't jibe with what you remember, you don't have to lock horns. Realize that both of you probably unwittingly harbor warped information in this shared memory, and resign yourself to never fully knowing the truth of what actually happened.

8

Tip of the Tongue

The other day, I couldn't come up with the name of the actor who played Tony Soprano in the HBO series *The Sopranos*. I knew I knew his name, but I couldn't bring it to mind. I knew that he had died unexpectedly while vacationing in Italy. The character of his wife, Carmela, was played by Edie Falco. He was in that lovely movie with Julia Louis-Dreyfus. I could picture him in my mind's eye. I could hear the sound of his voice. I went through the alphabet, searching for the first letter. *A?* Anthony? No, that's his character's name, not his real name. *J?* That feels right. John? Jack? Jerry? No, it's not any of those.

I *knew* his name was stored somewhere in my brain, and I felt vaguely close, but I couldn't produce it. I could retrieve so many other details about him, I felt I had to be in the right neural neighborhood. When I was in college, in the days before the Internet and when research required a trip to the library, certain overly competitive and unscrupulous students would sometimes obtain whatever information was needed from a bound periodical and then hide it to prevent other students from completing the assignment. Searching for Tony Soprano's real name in the circuits of my mind felt like searching the spines of the periodicals in my college library, staring at the empty slice of space on the shelf where the information I needed should be. The question knocked around in my head for hours, nagging me, obsessed with retrieving the answer. Distracted and feeling relentlessly harassed, I finally gave up and googled it.

ACTOR WHO PLAYED TONY SOPRANO
James Gandolfini

That's it! Sweet relief.

One of the most common experiences of memory failure is known as blocking or tip of the tongue (TOT). You're trying to come up with a word, most often a person's name, a city, a movie title, or the name of a book. You know you know the elusive word or phrase, but you cannot for the life of you retrieve it on demand. This blocked word is not forgotten. It's stored somewhere in your brain, hiding like a naughty dog that won't come when called. But you temporarily can't produce it.

Why does this happen? All words have neural representations and associated connections in your brain. Some neurons store the visual aspects of words—what they look like as printed letters. Other neurons store the word's conceptual information—what the word means, every sensory perception and emotion associated with it, any past experience you've had with it. Others are in charge of phonological information. These neurons hold what the word sounds like when spoken and are necessary for the verbal pronunciation of the word, either aloud or in your head.

Blocking can occur when there is only partial or weak activation of the neurons that connect to the word you're looking for. *What's her name? I can tell you it begins with an* L *but nothing else.* Without more neural activation, I get stuck there.

It can also happen when there is insufficient activation between the stored information about the word and the spelling or sound of that word, which is why I could come up with so much information about the actor who played Tony Soprano but I couldn't produce his name. It was on the tip of my tongue, but the name wouldn't come out of my mouth. I couldn't speak it.

A third to half of these instances typically resolve on their own. The word suddenly pops into consciousness sometime later. You're in the shower, and—poof!—the word comes to mind. Or you're in bed trying to fall asleep, and bam! James Gandolfini. Sometimes, you just bump into a retrieval cue that happens to be strong enough to trigger the activation of the word.

Relief can also come from outside assistance. You ask someone who offers the answer, or you google it as I did to remember who played Tony Soprano. You recognize the answer immediately. *Yes, that's it!*

During a TOT experience, we sometimes get a sneak peek of the word in question by way of the first letter or the number of syllables. We often experience a partial retrieval, these encouraging, yet wimpy hints. *I know it begins with a* D. If you speak a romance language like Italian or Spanish, you might know that the word is masculine or feminine. You know it ends in the letter *a*.

You also might come up with a loosely related word, something similar in sound or meaning to the word you're desperately trying to find. Psychologists call these obliquely related words the *ugly sisters* of the target, and unfortunately, zeroing in on an ugly sister unwittingly makes the situation worse. These decoys cause you to shift your attention, enticing you to follow neural pathways that lead to them and not to the word you really want. Now every time you try to retrieve the word in question, all you can think of is the ugly sister.

This happened to me the other day. I forget why (oh the

irony), but I was trying to remember the name of a certain city in Florida. I knew I knew it, but I couldn't find the word. I drew a blank. But not entirely.

It's near Miami. It begins with a B*? I think it begins with* B. *Is it Boca Raton? No, that's not it.*

Thirty minutes later, I still couldn't come up with it, and still the only city I could produce was Boca Raton. I felt frustrated, impatient, and uncomfortable.

Come on, brain. What's the name of that city?

Boca Raton.

No, stop saying that. That's not it.

I couldn't get any neurons other than "Boca Raton" to raise their hands. Unable to coax or threaten the answer into my consciousness, I finally gave up and resorted to Google Maps. I searched south of Miami, and boom! There it was!

Key Biscayne.

Interestingly, Key Biscayne is a two-word city, just like Boca Raton. And Biscayne. There was the *B*. Boca Raton was the ugly sister, capturing my attention, diverting it away from the neural pathways that would lead to Key Biscayne. I was deep in the wrong rabbit hole. The ugly sister effect also explains why the right word can sometimes bubble to the surface, seemingly out of nowhere, once you've stopped trying to find it. By calling off the hunt, my brain could stop perseverating on the wrong neural target, giving the correct set of neurons a chance to be activated.

Here's another example. My boyfriend Joe and I were talking about a colleague of his who is an avid surfer. I asked, "What's the name of that famous surfer? Lance?"

Joe said, "No, it's not Lance."

But he couldn't come up with it, either. Later, he told me that "Lance" sent his mind to Lance Armstrong, the cyclist. This was the ugly sister. Joe knew Lance Armstrong wasn't the answer, but his brain activity kept cycling through Lance's neighborhood, stubbornly and repeatedly searching the wrong set of neurons. His attention and recall were seduced by this ugly sister, which was interfering with his ability to find the real answer. If I hadn't offered my incorrect guess, Joe's brain might have found the surfer straight away.

"No, he's married to Gabrielle Reece, the volleyball player," he said.

I agreed, but this cue wasn't strong enough to unlock the surfer's name for either of us. Both of us were stumped, stuck in an uncomfortable TOT state. A few minutes later, Joe blurted out, "Laird Hamilton!"

What happened in Joe's brain that allowed him to find the answer? How did he free himself from the magnetism of the decoy and escape that TOT predicament? We can't know for sure (even he doesn't know), but it's likely that the right combination and number of associations were activated, accumulating enough strength to leave the ugly sister's spell and activate retrieval of the target word.

Even though my brain couldn't initially produce the name of the surfer, it did find the correct first letter. And although my brain couldn't recall Laird Hamilton's name, it immediately recognized that Laird was the name I was searching for when Joe said it. When you're in a TOT state and the target word is presented, you don't wonder if it's the right answer or need some time to consider it or fact-check. You call off the hunt right there. Hallelujah.

I could give you many additional personal TOT examples, especially instances of blocking on a person's name, because this is the most frequent kind of memory retrieval failure for all of us. And it's normal. Being in a TOT state does not mean you have Alzheimer's. Read that sentence again so it sinks in. The average twenty-five-year-old experiences several TOTs per week. But young people don't sweat them, in part because memory loss, Alzheimer's, old age, and mortality are nowhere on their radars. And because young people today have been tethered to devices since childhood, they don't hesitate to outsource the job to their smartphones. They seldom suffer in TOT misery for hours (or even minutes) like their parents, who stubbornly insist on recalling the missing name the old-school way, without the assistance of Google.

The frequency of TOTs we experience does normally increase with age, probably because of a decrease in our brain's processing speed. But we *notice* them more when we're older because aging and Alzheimer's are more immediate realities and possibilities. If you have Alzheimer's disease in your family, you're likely to find that word blocking feels all the more alarming and personal. Convinced these episodes are pathological, we become increasingly afraid of our retrieval failures when we're older. While they're admittedly frustrating, they're probably no cause for a visit to the neurologist. The elusive word will eventually pop into consciousness. And if you can't stand the discomfort for one more second, there's no shame or punishment for using Google.

Many people worry that if they use Google to find their blocked words, then they're contributing to the problem and actually worsening their already-weakening memory. They consider Google a high-tech crutch that's going to ruin their memories. This belief is misinformed. Looking up the name of the actor who played Tony Soprano doesn't weaken my memory's ability whatsoever. Similarly, suffering through the mental pain and insisting on coming up with the word on my own doesn't make my memory stronger or come with any trophies for my doing so. You don't have to be a memory martyr. You are not more likely to experience fewer TOTs, resolve future TOTs faster, better remember where you put your keys, remember to take your heart medication tonight, or prevent Alzheimer's if you can retrieve Tony Soprano's name without Google.

TOTs are a normal glitch in memory retrieval, a by-product

of how our brains are organized. You wear glasses if your eyes need help seeing. You can use Google if a word is stuck on the tip of your tongue.

In the hierarchy of Things People Tend to Forget, proper names are significantly more vulnerable to blocking than are common words. Forgetting people's names is an entirely normal and frequent phenomenon and is not an early sign of Alzheimer's. Here's why.

Let's imagine that I show you and a friend a photograph of a man's face. I tell you that the man in the picture is a baker. I tell your friend that the last name of the man in the picture is Baker. A couple of days later, I show each of you the same photograph and ask if you can remember anything about the man in the picture. You are much more likely to remember baker than your friend is to remember Baker.

But wait. You and your friend saw the exact same photograph and heard the exact same word. Why would the same information be better remembered if the word *baker* is stored in memory as an occupation rather than as a person's name?

This phenomenon is known as the *Baker/baker paradox*. Even if you don't know anyone who is a baker, baking as a profession is probably connected to many associations, synapses, and neural circuits in your brain. When you are told that the guy in the photograph is a baker, you might visualize him wearing a white hat and an apron. You could picture him holding a rolling pin or a wooden spoon. You might think about the fresh-baked bread you had with dinner last night. You might remember the bakery you used to go to as a kid and how much you loved its cinnamon doughnuts. You might picture and imagine the smell and taste of apple pie.

If instead you're told that the photograph is of a man named Baker, unless you personally know someone with that last name, what do you imagine? Nothing. Baker as a last name is an abstract concept, a neurological cul-de-sac. Because the name isn't connected to any information in your brain other than what you see in the photograph you're looking at, his name is much more difficult to remember. The neural architecture that supports baker as a profession is stronger because it has many more elaborate connections and possible neural roads for activation—words, memories, associations, and other meaning—cues that can trigger the word *baker* in response to "Who is this guy?" If you liken memory retrieval to a Google search, you'll get many more hits for "baker" than for "Baker."

The Baker/baker paradox also explains why so many of us are bad at remembering names but not at recalling other details about a person. When I see a woman I've met before, I might easily remember that she's a physician, that she's from New York City, and that she vacationed last year in New Zealand. But for the life of me, I cannot recall her name. Is it Sharon? Susan? Stephanie? I can't remember.

Thankfully, an understanding of this paradox also gives us a strategy for better remembering people's names and reducing the frequency of these TOT episodes. Because proper names are, by neurological nature, so much harder to remember, you can assist your memory by turning your Bakers into bakers. Mr. Baker has no associations in your brain, but baker does. Connect them! Imagine Mr. Baker in the picture wearing a white hat and an apron and with flour on his face. He holds a spatula in his hand, and he is baking chocolate chip cookies.

In the example of the woman from New York, the physician who vacationed in New Zealand and whose name I couldn't remember, let's say her name is Sarah Green. I could picture *Sarah* Jessica Parker wearing an I Heart NYC T-shirt, donning a stethoscope, listening to the heartbeat of a sheep on a lush *green* field in New Zealand. Now I've linked the abstract name Sarah Green to a number of elaborate, visual, colorful, and even strange details. Next time I see Sarah Green, I have a much better chance of engaging the activity of neurons that are connected and that will lead to the recall of her name.

Now that you're hopefully not terrified of TOTs, and you know that blocking is an annoyingly frequent but normal type of retrieval failure, let's see if I can make you experience one. Following is a list of ten questions. Some you'll be able to answer quickly and easily. For some, you'll know that you don't know the answer. This isn't a memory failure. You simply don't have the information in your brain. For others, you'll know you know the answer, but you can't produce it.

---

answer instantly. Neurologically, recognition is always easier than recall.

Still stumped? It's in your brain. Keep looking. Or you can wait and see if the answer pops into your consciousness later. Or, because I appreciate how uncomfortable being in a TOT state can be and because I'm kind and mostly because I want your full attention on what you're going to read in the next chapter, here are the answers to the ten questions listed on the opposite page: Brasília, Freddie Mercury, 186,282 miles per second, Stephen King, Rome, Venus, Woody Guthrie, ask your mom, Lisa Kudrow, Vincent van Gogh.

Feel better?

9

Don't Forget to Remember

I need to remember to call my mother,
schedule a doctor's appointment,
take my allergy pill,
buy milk,
take out the trash tomorrow morning,
text my brother,
drop off the dry cleaning,
move the laundry from the washer to the dryer,
reply to Ken's e-mail,
meet Greg for coffee at 11:00,
pick up my daughter at 3:00,
go to the bank before it closes.

Prospective memory is your memory for what you need to do later. This kind of memory is a bit like mental time travel. You're creating an intention for your future you. This is your brain's to-do list, a memory to be recalled at a future time and place. And it is fraught with forgetting. In fact, prospective memory is so poorly supported by our neural circuitry and so steeped in failure, it can almost be thought of as a kind of forgetting rather than a kind of memory.

For a prospective memory to be remembered and not forgotten, the intention or the action that needs to be performed later needs first to be encoded into memory now. This step rarely presents a problem. I need to remember to book my daughter's flight home from college before I go to bed tonight. There. I've asked my brain to remember to do this task. It's in there.

The second step is where I'm likely to run into all kinds of trouble. I have to remember to remember this task. And generally speaking, our brains are terrible at remembering to remember. Not just aging brains. All brains. The memory of that intention (book my daughter's flight home) needs to be retrieved in the future (before bed), twelve hours from now. Because booking a flight for my daughter isn't a well-ingrained, habitual pre-bedtime task like brushing my teeth, unless I create at least one specific cue that will trigger the recall of "booking my daughter's flight before I go to bed," I am likely to forget to make the reservation.

Prospective memories rely on external cues to trigger their recall. Those cues can be time based—at a certain time or after a certain time interval, remember to do something. *At 2:50, you need to remember to go pick up your kid at school.* Or they can be event based—when a particular thing happens, remember to do something. *When you see Diane, ask her if she can pick up your kid at school.*

But because we sometimes set up not-so-great cues or miss the cues when we're supposed to notice them, this kind of memory is highly susceptible to failure. We forget to do what we intended to do. A lot. Prospective memory is that flaky friend who likes to make plans with you to meet for drinks but half the time is a no-show. This kind of capricious, absent-minded forgetting plagues most of us on a daily basis. We forget to buy toothpaste, call our mothers, and return that overdue book to the library.

See if any of the following situations feel familiar to you. The questions below are taken from the Prospective and Retrospective Memory Questionnaire. Rate your answers as 5 (very often), 4 (quite often), 3 (sometimes), 2 (rarely), or 1 (never).

1. Do you decide to do something in a few minutes' time and then forget to do it?

2. Do you fail to do something you were supposed to do a few minutes later even though it's there in front of you, like take a pill or turn off the kettle?
3. Do you forget appointments if you are not prompted by someone else or by a reminder such as a calendar or a diary?
4. Do you forget to buy something you planned to buy, like a birthday card, even when you see the shop?
5. Do you intend to take something with you, before leaving a room or going out, but minutes later leave it behind, even though it's there in front of you?
6. Do you fail to mention or give something to a visitor that you were asked to pass on?
7. If you tried to contact a friend or a relative who was out, would you forget to try again later?
8. Do you forget to tell someone something you had meant to mention a few minutes ago?

How did you do? My score was 25. I didn't answer 1 (never) or 2 (rarely) for any of the questions.

Marketing companies take advantage of our prospective-memory vulnerabilities all the time. You join an online exercise program, download a meditation app, or subscribe to a magazine for a free thirty-day trial, fully planning to cancel or unsubscribe if you find that you don't use or like it. It turns out that you don't love the workout, you can't get into the habit of meditating, and you don't read any of the magazine articles past the first couple of days, but on your next credit card statement, you see that you've been charged $99 for the year. You forgot to unsubscribe.

In 1997, researchers looked at prospective memory and aging in one thousand adults aged thirty-five to eighty. Everyone in the study was screened for various health, socioeconomic, and cognitive information. But here was the real test. At the beginning of the screening session, each subject was asked to remind the experimenter to sign a form when the session was over, which would be about two hours later. How do you think everyone did?

Only about half of the thirty-five- to forty-year-olds remembered to tell the experimenter to sign the form. Surprisingly, the forty-five-year-olds did the best, with 75 percent remembering what to do. (The authors of the study were perplexed about why this age cohort performed significantly better than did folks a decade younger, and offered no compelling arguments or hypotheses about why.) But performance went steadily downhill from there. Less than half of the fifty- to sixty-year-olds remembered to ask the experimenter to sign the form. About 35 percent of the sixty-five- to seventy-year-olds and only about 20 percent of the seventy-five- to eighty-year-olds remembered.

What happens if the experimenter were to help by providing an additional cue? Let's say the subjects forgot what they were supposed to do and didn't ask the experimenter to sign the form at the end of the session. What if the experimenter then offered a hint? "Is there anything left for you to do?" Wink, wink. Across all ages, this prompt improved recall, but still, no age achieved 100 percent. And from age sixty-five on, less than half remembered to remember.

Maybe we're all more prone to forget to remember the little things, the mundane tasks that aren't life-and-death, intentions that aren't monumental. Maybe you would place more money on your prospective-memory prowess if what you needed to remember were critically important to you. Are prospective memories for high-priority tasks immune to forgetting?

Not at all.

On Saturday October 16, 1999, the world's most famous cellist, Yo-Yo Ma, climbed into a New York City yellow cab, rode about twenty minutes to the Peninsula Hotel, paid the fare, and got out. Moments after the taxi drove away, he remembered what he had forgotten. He had left his 266-year-old $2.5 million cello in the trunk. How could this have happened? That expensive, rare, exquisite instrument was the most important thing in Ma's life.

He later explained he was tired and in a rush, and so he was probably distracted and not at his cognitive best. But the biggest reason why Yo-Yo Ma forgot his cello? The cello case—that gigantic unmistakable cue—was missing from view. The prospective memory—remember to take the cello with you when you get out of the cab—failed to be activated without a cue to trigger it as he stepped out of the car. Out of sight, out of mind. To his profound relief, police found and returned the cello to Yo-Yo Ma later that day.

In a similar story, soloist Lynn Harrell left his seventeenth-century $4 million Stradivarius cello in the trunk of another New York City cab. His cello was also, thankfully, retrieved. What's going on here? Are cellists who are in possession of pricey antique instruments unusually susceptible to prospective forgetting?

They're not. Prospective memory is unreliable in all of us. Even surgeons. In 2013, the Joint Commission, a U.S. health-care safety watchdog, reported 772 surgical instruments forgotten and left inside patients over the previous eight years. A surgeon who removed a tumor from a man in Wisconsin forgot to remove a thirteen-inch retractor before closing him up. A six-inch metal clamp was left inside the intestine of a man from California. Scissors, scalpels, sponges, and gloves have been forgotten and left inside people's bodies an alarming number of times.

Remembering to retrieve your priceless cello from the trunk of a cab or to remove a foot-long surgical instrument from the abdominal cavity of another person is kind of a big deal. These examples can't be like forgetting to buy bread or take out the trash. And, yet, they are, in fact, the same. Without the right cue or cues in place at the right time, and without your attention available to notice those cues, you will forget what you're supposed to remember.

Prospective memory is challenging for people of all ages (does your teenager ever remember to shut off the bedroom light when leaving the room?) and occupations (certainly for surgeons and cellists). Still, we tend to unfairly judge and be judged for this kind of universally experienced absentmindedness. If a colleague forgets to show up for an important meeting or your teenager forgets to turn off the oven after baking cookies, you might very well interpret these prospective-memory lapses as signs of carelessness, poor character, unreliability, irresponsibility, or even a possible symptom of Alzheimer's. But the blame shouldn't point to a neurodegenerative disease or a lack of character. Forgetting to bring the gift, which is wrapped and ready and sitting on your kitchen table, to the birthday party you just arrived at is more likely due to a lack of proper cues than to character. To err is human, especially if you're relying on your prospective memory.

Which is why we need to help it . . .

MAKE TO-DO LISTS. We can create external aids for our prospective memory. If you begin to require better lighting while squinting to read the printed words on menus held at arm's length or if you keep increasing the font size on your phone, what do you do? You get glasses. If your eyes fail to see the world perfectly, you recruit help from an external aid called glasses to correct for this shortcoming.

Think of to-do lists as glasses for your prospective memory. There is no shame in a list. Don't trust that you'll remember later what you plan now. You probably won't. Write it down, people.

I recently went to the grocery store to buy milk so that I could make waffles for my kids. I drove to the store, I bought a bunch of things, and I came home—with no milk. And I only realized that I had forgotten the milk when I walked into the kitchen and saw the waffle maker on the counter. Next time, unless I want to carry the cue (the waffle maker) with me to the store, I should make a list. I just have to remember to bring the list with me.

And it's not enough to create to-do lists. You have to check them. The routine of checking a list is part of the solution for those surgeons who, because they are human and have unreliable prospective memories, risk forgetting to remove their surgical instruments from the patient's body before closing it up. They now have checklists that, when paid attention to, enable them to account for the whereabouts of every single piece of equipment used during an operation. Likewise, airplane pilots don't rely on their fickle prospective memories to remember to lower the wheels before landing the plane. Thankfully, they use checklists.

ENTER THE INFORMATION INTO YOUR CALENDAR. The retention intervals for prospective memory can be challenging. If you have to remember to bring a check to your daughter's dance class next week, holding this intention in your conscious awareness for the next seven days is both impractical and impossible.

So, just as you do with to-do lists, you want to externalize your brain's calendar. Don't count on your unreliable prospective memory to remember that you need to attend a meeting tomorrow at 4:00. Your brain might forget and get you in trouble. Make a habit of entering into your calendar anything you need to do in the future. And then make a habit of either checking your calendar many times a day or, if you're using a smartphone or computer, setting alarms or alert messages that will remind you to look at your calendar now.

Ping! It's 3:50. You have a meeting at 4:00. Go!

BE SPECIFIC ABOUT YOUR PLAN. Tying a white string around your finger only tells you that you need to remember to do something. Unless you need to buy more string, this cue is too nonspecific to reliably lead you to the memory you're searching for.

And don't tell your prospective memory, "I want to exercise later today." You haven't built in any specific cues to trigger activation of this intention. What kind of exercise? Where do you need to be to exercise? When are you going to exercise? Let's face it. You're not going to remember to exercise today.

Instead, tell yourself, "I'm going to go to yoga at noon." Now you have what psychologists call an *implementation intention*. Place your yoga mat by the front door. There's your visible cue. Enter "yoga at noon" into your calendar, and set a reminder alert to go off at 11:45 because you know it takes ten minutes to drive there.

Namaste.

USE PILLBOXES. Forgetting to take your medication is one of the most common and problematic prospective-memory failures. Luckily, you can overcome this challenge by using simple pillboxes and reminders. Pillboxes organize your medications into individual sections for each day of the week (or even for several times per day if needed). Setting calendar alerts or using a pill reminder app can serve as the cue that sends you to your pillbox. This strategy also helps with the episodic memory failure of *Did I already take my pills today?* You can go to the pillbox and see if the section for Tuesday is empty. Two memory birds, one pillbox stone. But wait, what day is it?

PLACE YOUR CUES IN IMPOSSIBLE-TO-MISS LOCATIONS. Let's say I bought a bottle of wine to bring to a friend's dinner party tomorrow night. The bottle is in a brown paper bag on my kitchen counter. Unless I add "bring wine bottle" to my to-do list or add "bring wine bottle" to my calendar for tomorrow night, and unless I happen to notice the brown-bagged bottle on my counter before leaving home, there's a good chance I will show up at my friend's house empty-handed.

My boyfriend prevents this kind of prospective-memory failure by placing near the front door anything that needs to come with us. Need to bring a bottle of wine to the party? He puts it on the floor, in front of the door. Don't forget to bring the tickets for the concert. On the floor, in front of the door. I need to remember to mail this letter. On the floor, in front of the door. We would literally have to trip over the items to be remembered just to leave the house.

You don't need to use the front door, but this method is sound practice. Make sure your cues are in the right place for you to notice them in time for you to do what you intended. If you need to take your medication at night before bed, place your pillbox next to your toothbrush and not hidden away inside a cabinet, where you can't see it.

BE AWARE IF YOUR ROUTINE HAS BEEN DISRUPTED. Many of us use some part of our daily routine as a prospective-memory cue. Getting ready for bed prompts you to remember to brush your teeth. You take your daily medications with coffee and breakfast, so a bagel and a dark roast are your cues reminding you to take your heart medication.

But be mindful if your daily routine deviates or becomes temporarily disrupted, because the cues you're relying on may have shifted or disappeared. If you skip breakfast today because you're late for an early appointment, will you forget to take your heart medication? Any time your day derails, take a moment to look for any prospective-memory to-do tasks that may have been coupled to the activity that moved or didn't happen.

And the next time you're in a taxi or an Uber, before you step one foot out of that car, think, "Did I leave my cello in the trunk?"

10

This Too Shall Pass

List everything you did today from the moment you woke up. Really sit with this exercise for a minute (and if you're reading this at 8:00 A.M. and haven't done much of anything yet today, list everything you did yesterday). Think about all the sensory experiences, what you did, who you were with, the weather, what you wore, what you ate and drank, where you were, what you learned, how you felt. Remember everything you can from today.

Now do this same exercise for exactly one week ago. One month ago. This day, last year. While you might remember quite a lot from today or even yesterday, you probably recall less and less as you look back. If you're like me, you're staring at a blank page for this day last year.

What happened to the memories of all those experiences and pieces of information?

Time. Time happened.

The number one archenemy of the memories you've created and stored is time. It's not enough to pay attention to an experience, pluck some pieces of sensory information and emotion from it, bind them together into a singular memory, and then store that memory through alterations in synaptic connections between the neurons that were originally activated by that experience. If you don't revisit the memory, if it just sits on your brain's cortical shelf like an old trophy collecting dust, that memory will erode with the passage of time.

But does it fade to black? Over time, if a memory isn't activated, will it eventually be erased, or will there always be a trace? Could the seemingly lost details of this day last year be revived if your brain got the right prompt? Would you recognize the details of this day last year if I presented them to you? Or has that memory completely decayed, the information no longer existing in your brain? Have those synaptic connections—that memory—literally disappeared?

These questions were first asked and answered scientifically by Hermann Ebbinghaus in 1885. In trying to figure out how quickly we forget what we learn, he created 2,300 nonsense one-syllable "words" like these:

wid
zof
laj
nud
kep

So that he could pronounce them, he put them all in the form of consonant-vowel-consonant. But these fabricated words were meaningless, so he couldn't form any obvious associations. He memorized lists of these made-up words and then tested his ability to remember them after short retention intervals (immediately afterward, a few minutes later, an hour later) and long ones (the next day, the next week).

His findings aren't particularly surprising. The longer the retention interval between learning and recall, the more he forgot. His big conclusion—memory is transient. It eventually fades.

In his own case, Ebbinghaus found that forgetting occurred quite rapidly at first. He forgot almost half of the nonwords he had memorized after only twenty minutes. But after twenty-four hours, forgetting leveled off to a retention rate of about 25 percent. Called the *Ebbinghaus forgetting curve,* this pattern is generally what happens to unsupported memory over time. Without deliberate attempts or strategies to retain what you learn, you will forget most of what you experience almost right away. The steep, dramatic, and prompt decline of memory then levels off. What little you still remember after that initial data dump seems to stay with you.

Say you learned a language in high school and haven't spoken it since. Because you stopped using it, you lost most of what you had learned within the following year, but then the forgetting leveled off. And what remains of that language in your memory can be stable for the next fifty years. I took three years of Latin in high school. Other than a framed diploma or two, I haven't looked at this language since I was sixteen. It's decades later, and I still know how to conjugate "to be"—*sum, es, est, sumus, estis, sunt*—from memory. But I don't remember much else. Without use, repetition, or significance, most of our memories fade quickly. Over time, if any memory remains, it appears to be permanently stored.

So according to Ebbinghaus and his forgetting curve, although the information we encode into memory degrades rapidly with the passage of time, it doesn't entirely disappear. Also in support of memory's not being utterly obliterated by time, Ebbinghaus was the first to demonstrate memory savings. Say it initially took him ten attempts to remember a list of nonsense words with no mistakes. He then waited and waited, until at last, he had forgotten the entire list. When he later went to relearn that same list, he needed only five attempts to memorize it with no mistakes. So even when he eventually couldn't consciously recall a single nonword from the list, the list wasn't in fact entirely forgotten. His brain hadn't gone back to the way it was before he initially learned the nonwords. Trace memories of those nonwords remained, making it easier to activate and relearn the list.

But there is also evidence that memories can be physiologically erased. More recent studies have shown that if the collection of synapses representing a memory isn't activated over time, the connections will be physically pruned away. If dormant for too long, neurons will literally retract their anatomical, electrochemical connections with other neurons. The connections, and consequently the memory contained in those connections, will no longer exist.

We've all experienced both scenarios. I took Italian in seventh and eighth grade and, until recently, hadn't studied or spoken it since. If you had asked me to speak the days of the week in Italian, I would have come up totally blank. I would have claimed and believed that I had completely forgotten this information. But if you had then recited *lunedì*, *martedì* . . . this might have been enough of a prompt for me to blurt out *mercoledì*, *giovedì*, *venerdì*, *sabato*, *domenica*. Whoa! Where did that come from? Those Italian days of the week still existed as a memory in my brain, and I didn't even know it!

Alternatively, sometimes, no matter how many cues someone offers, you just can't remember what you once apparently knew. Recently, a friend made a reference to the Peloponnesian War. I know I studied this war in some history class when I was in high school. I probably crammed for the test and remembered the information long enough to spit it out on the day of the exam. But then, because I really didn't care about this war at all, in accordance with Ebbinghaus's forgetting curve for meaningless information, I promptly forgot most of what I had memorized. And because I became a neuroscientist and not a historian and never revisited what I learned about the Peloponnesian War, whatever memories persisted after that exam were probably physiologically deleted over time. No matter what or how many details my friend shared about this war, nothing rang a bell. I think those neural connections were pruned away.

Whether a memory ultimately fades, either to some degree or entirely, is influenced by what you do with the information once it is housed in your brain. There are two main ways to resist the effects of time on memory: repetition and meaning.

If you want to retain the information you've managed to store in your brain, keep activating it. Revisit the information again and again. Reminisce, rehearse, and repeat. You can significantly decrease the amount of memory that will be lost to time by repetition to the point of overlearning. In other words, learn until you self-test at 100 percent, and then keep studying. Rehearse *past* mastery. To this day, I can recite Macbeth's "Tomorrow and tomorrow and tomorrow" soliloquy by William Shakespeare from memory and without error because I overlearned that sucker in eleventh grade.

Have you ever been in your car when a song comes on the radio that you haven't heard in twenty years, but you instantly know all the lyrics? You start singing along and don't miss a word. Most likely, twenty years ago, when the song was popular, you heard and sang it many times a day. The radio stations overplayed it, and so you overlearned it. When it comes to saving your memories, repetition is a mighty warrior in the battle against time.

But maybe you want to forget something. Let's say your spouse cheated on you, and you got divorced. Want to forget the sordid details and the heartache you're feeling? Stop repeating the story of what happened. Stop going over the details with your friends and in your thoughts. Don't overlearn the experience. If you can find the discipline to leave those memories alone, they will eventually fade. And while you will always remember that your ex cheated on you, the emotional elements of that memory can gradually decay if left alone. It is through the erosion of memory that time heals all wounds.

The other main way to protect memory from time is to add meaning. If I give you three nonsense words to memorize—*grudelon, micadeltere, fidiklud*—you're likely to forget them rather quickly. If instead I ask you to memorize three real words—*ukulele, microphone, rainbow*—you'll have no problem remembering them. Because this collection of letters has meaning, your brain can assemble them into a meaningful story.

> The woman sang "Somewhere Over the Rainbow" into the microphone while playing the ukulele.

Your brain loves meaning. If you take what you want to remember and wrap a story around it, making associations with what you already know and care about, or if you place it in a special moment in your life's narrative, you will make that memory resistant to forgetting. And if a memory is meaningful to you, you're more likely to think about it, share it, use it, and reminisce about it. In this way, meaningful memories are often repeated and thus become even stronger. Ebbinghaus's nonsense words, quickly forgotten, were meaningless. His forgetting curve takes on an entirely different shape if the information we want to retain has meaning.

Think of a movie that you watched recently but that you didn't love. For me, this would be *La La Land*. How many details about that movie can you remember? *It starred Emma Stone and Ryan Gosling.* What was the plot? *I don't really remember what it was about. I know they sang and danced.* Can you remember whom you saw it with? *No.* Did you eat popcorn or any other snacks while watching the movie? *I don't remember.* What day of the week was it? *No idea.* Were you on a plane or at your local theater, or did you watch it at home? *I was either on a plane or at home.* Can you remember any of the dialogue verbatim? *Definitely no.*

Why can't I remember that movie or this day last year?

Neither the movie nor the day contained enough meaning to stick around. This day last year was probably a routine string of Starbucks, writing, lunch, errands, after-school activities, dinner, repeatedly telling my children to go brush their teeth, and going to sleep—too mundane and similar to hundreds of other days. Unless that breakfast, that list of words, that conversation, that chapter in the book, that Starbucks chai latte, that movie were especially meaningful (and therefore meaningful enough to be revisited, shared, repeated, reread, and even overlearned), time would have dissolved those memories entirely or faded them into vague bits and pieces—the bottom of the forgetting curve. *La La Land* didn't do it for me, and so a year later, I can barely recall anything about it.

Now think of a movie that you loved when you saw it, and ask yourself the same questions. Notice the difference in your answers, both the quantity and the quality.

I saw *A Star Is Born* last year with Joe and my friend Sara at the Boston Common movie theater. Sara and I ate popcorn. We walked there. It was October. Sara sat on my left, and Joe on my right, and we all sat right of center, about a dozen rows from the front. I loved this movie. The emotional impact stayed with me for weeks. Sara and I texted back and forth about it, about unconditional love and addiction and vulnerability. I sang along with the songs from the soundtrack on Spotify, and I listened to a podcast interview between Oprah and Bradley Cooper about the film. Unlike my impression of

11

Fuggedaboutit

Solomon Shereshevsky, known in neuroscience and psychology texts as "S., the Man Who Could Not Forget," had an extraordinary memory. Russian psychologist Alexander Luria tested and retested Shereshevsky's ability to remember over a span of thirty years. Shereshevsky could memorize massively long lists of numbers or nonsensical information, pages of poetry in foreign languages that he didn't speak, and complex scientific formulas that he didn't understand. Even more astounding, he could recall these lists in order and without error when Luria retested him years later.

Sounds like an amazing superpower, yes? But Shereshevsky's extraordinary ability to remember astonishing volumes of information came at a price. He felt burdened by excessive and often irrelevant information and had enormous difficulty filtering, prioritizing, and forgetting what he didn't want or need. His inability to forget was at times a profound handicap in daily life.

We tend to vilify forgetting. We cast it as the bad guy in the epic battle against everyone's favorite hero, Remembering. But forgetting isn't always a regrettable sign of aging, a pathological symptom of dementia, a shameful failure, a maladaptive problem to solve, or even accidental. Remembering today the details of what happened yesterday isn't always beneficial. Sometimes, we want to forget what we know.

Forgetting is quite important; it helps us function every day in all kinds of ways. It's advantageous for us to get rid of any unnecessary, irrelevant, interfering, or even painful memories that can potentially distract us or cause us to make mistakes or feel miserable. Sometimes we need to forget one thing in order to pay attention to—and remember—another, and so in this way, forgetting can *facilitate* better memory.

We also tend to think of forgetting as our default setting. Unless you actively do something to remember some piece of information, your brain will automatically forget it. Easily. And if you're over fifty, too easily. We forget without trying. We forget what that woman just said because we didn't pay enough attention. We forget to pick up the dry cleaning because we didn't create strong enough relevant cues. We can't recall what we learned about the Industrial Revolution in eleventh grade because too much time has elapsed without periodic recall. We are the powerless, passive victims of forgetting. It happens to us. But forgetting can also be artful—active, deliberate, motivated, targeted, and desirable.

For example, I travel a lot when I'm on a book or speaking tour and can be in a different city every night. Being able to rattle off the last four hotel room numbers I stayed in might be an impressive feat, but it's actually better for me to have forgotten last night's room number when I find myself in the elevator at the next hotel. If every room number I've stayed in for the past four nights enters my consciousness when I step into that elevator, I'll probably get confused and not know which button to push. I want to forget each hotel room number as soon as I check out. An intelligent memory system not only remembers information but also actively forgets whatever is no longer useful.

Similarly, with two young kids and a college-aged daughter who typically comes and goes with several other similarly sized, endlessly snacking friends, I'm at the grocery store many times a week. Every time I push a carriage full of bagged groceries out of the store, I have to remember, *Where did I park my car?* If in this moment, I retrieve where I parked last month and last week and yesterday, I'll have too much irrelevant information online, and I won't know where to go. I only want to retrieve where I parked today. And so forgetting all those previous spaces is a good idea. Similarly, I'll want to forget where I parked today after I return to my car so I don't confuse the memory of that location with where I'll park tomorrow.

Forgetting this kind of routine detail isn't a deficit we need to fix or worry about. Imagine a list of your daily tasks scrawled on a whiteboard—showering, getting dressed, drinking coffee, eating breakfast, commuting, parking, and so on. That whiteboard is crowded with perceptions, information, and experiences by the end of each day. Forgetting the mundane and inconsequential will wipe the whiteboard clean, creating space for a new day and thereby facilitating the retention and recall of what you want to remember next.

But it ain't always easy. We tend to think of remembering as the challenge, but forgetting can be difficult, too. I changed the password on my Netflix account about a month ago, and for the next several weeks, I couldn't get my fingers to stop typing the old password when prompted by the cursor. My muscle memory for the old password persisted, interfering with the retrieval of the new memory for the new password—and the formation of that new muscle memory for my fingers. I needed to forget the old password and replace it with the new.

If I could leave the memory for that old password alone, time would eventually weaken and fade it. But there's the problem. I can't leave it alone. I keep activating and reinforcing the strength of the memory for the old password every time I inadvertently type it.

While much of the forgetting that we experience tends to be accidental and passive—due to the natural decay of the biological connections or a lack of regular retrieval—there are, at every phase of the memory process, ways to actively forget what we don't want to keep. As described earlier, the first step in creating a memory is encoding an experience or information. You have to both perceive and pay attention to create a memory. So one way of intentionally forgetting is to not pay attention in the first place. Look away. Don't listen. Create a diversion. The information won't get encoded. This is the fingers-in-your-ears, la-la-la-I-can't-hear-you method of intentionally forgetting. Motivated redirection of attention is a powerful way to ensure that an experience or information won't be retained.

But let's say you paid attention and the information seeped into your brain. You can then consciously or unconsciously discard information and selectively forget during the consolidation process. For example, we tend to limit the consolidation of negative information about ourselves, and so this information is never stored long term. We sort out the unflattering stuff and forget about it.

In a fun study on positivity bias, psychologists gave subjects a fake personality test. Tests were "scored," and each subject was presented with the same fake result—a list of thirty-two personality traits describing the subject, some positive and some not so much. Subjects were later asked to recall as many of the traits as possible.

What did they remember? They recalled far more positive traits than negative *unless* they were told that the list of traits was about someone else. In that case, they remembered an equal number of positive and negative traits. We possess a positivity bias with respect to how we see ourselves. We tend to selectively consolidate and then remember the good qualities about ourselves and actively exclude and therefore forget the bad.

Now what if you want to forget a memory that was already consolidated and has made its way into long-term storage? In this case, you want to avoid exposure to the cues and context that will trigger its retrieval. Don't go there. Don't think about the memory or talk about it. Don't inadvertently rehearse it. If you catch yourself beginning to sing that annoying commercial jingle, stop singing. Cancel, cancel. Don't finish the song. Redirect your thoughts. Resist activating the neural circuitry of this unwanted memory, because every time you fully retrieve it, you will reinforce it. The more you're able to leave it alone, the more it will weaken and be forgotten.

Of course, this strategy is much easier said than done and is especially difficult for people who have experienced trauma. People with post-traumatic stress disorder (PTSD) can't stop retrieving, reliving, and reconsolidating unwanted memories, and unfortunately, these individuals unwittingly strengthen these memories with every unwelcome recall. Preventing the activation of even part of an unwanted memory—and especially the emotional aspects of the experience—can give time the chance to do its magic, allowing the memory to fade. But this can feel seemingly impossible to do. People with PTSD can't stop remembering the sexual assault, the car accident, the day in combat. They can't forget.

Another potential and possibly more promising approach to forgetting traumatic memories asks the person to continue to revisit the memory with the intention of introducing changes. As explained earlier, when we revisit a memory for something that happened, we can alter it, and then we reconsolidate and store version 2.0, essentially writing over the original. This memory revision is usually done unintentionally.

But what if we could artfully design version 2.0 so that the updated memory for what happened no longer contains trauma-inducing details? What if, under the guidance of a trained therapist, we could reformat painful memories by omitting the fear- and anxiety-inducing details during reconsolidation? By taking advantage of episodic memory's proclivity for editing, maybe painful memories could be replaced by kinder, gentler, emotionally neutral versions of what happened.

If you can't avoid the cues or context or revisiting a memory, in the words of Elsa from the movie *Frozen*, let it go. Tell your brain, "Forget about it. Don't keep this. Let it go"—and your brain might obey. Self-instruction can work and is thought to do so by both derailing consolidation before new memories are fully created and activating neural signaling programs that deliberately erase memories already formed.

Visualization can also help with self-directed requests to forget. Burdened with excessive information, Shereshevsky was desperate to rid his brain of unwanted, superfluous memories. He envisioned his unwelcome memories catching fire, the information going up in flames and smoke, nothing left but ash. Great imagery, but unfortunately for Shereshevsky, the memory remained stubbornly emblazoned in his brain.

Luckily, he persisted. He pictured the memory of what he wanted to forget as meaningless information drawn in white chalk on a blackboard. He then imagined erasing the image, wiping the chalkboard clean. This visualization worked. Through imagery and the intentional direction to remove a memory from conscious awareness, Shereshevsky, a man famous for remembering everything, was blessedly able to forget.

Swapping out clingy muscle memories like typing an old password or the habit of an incorrectly learned golf swing for new memories requires a different strategy. Because muscle memories are performed without conscious instruction, these memorized procedural skills will be impervious to conscious requests to take a hike. Instead, we replace our old password with a new one or an old golf swing with a better stroke in the same way that we learned the earlier version. Practice, practice, practice. Type that new password over and over until your fingers automatically prefer the 2.0 version. Keep swinging that club until the new motion becomes automatic, rewriting the muscle memory for how to swing a driver.

What mediates motivated forgetting? We don't really know. Although the neuroscience of intentional forgetting is still in its infancy, an eventual understanding of how the brain actively forgets may well give us better insight into neurological disorders and mental illnesses such as PTSD, depression, autism, schizophrenia, and addiction. In all of these conditions, an inability to forget memory-associated cues proves maladaptive.

So while we all want an amazing memory, we can't put all the onus and credit on remembering. An optimally functioning memory system involves a finely orchestrated balancing act between data storage and data disposal: remembering and forgetting. When performing optimally, memory doesn't remember everything. It retains what is meaningful and useful, and it discards what isn't. It keeps the signal and purges the noise. Our ability to forget is likely to be just as vital as is our ability to remember.

12

Normal Aging

Forgetting at any age is a normal part of human memory. We forget because we didn't pay attention, because we don't have the right cues or context, because what happened was routine or inconsequential, because we never practiced, because we didn't get enough sleep or are too stressed out, or because too much time has passed. But as we age, forgetting gets, well, older.

As you've aged, you've probably noticed some not-so-delightful changes in your body's appearance and performance. Your hair might be going gray, crow's-feet may be clawing at the corners of your eyes, and what appears to be a trench is forming between your eyebrows. You can no longer read the washing instructions on clothing tags without glasses, and your time on that annual 5K is probably a full minute slower than it was last year. Oh yeah, and your memory doesn't feel as powerful as it used to be. That might be putting it mildly.

Unpredictably sluggish, unreliable, and unresponsive, your memory may be acting like a bad employee—regularly late and unprepared for meetings, not answering the phone, and often caught asleep and drooling at its desk. Your memory didn't always act this way (or so you think you remember). It used to be really good at its job. But lately, not so much.

Your most common complaint: Your memory regularly struggles to fetch the word you're searching for. It may or may not be on the tip of your tongue. You wait in front of an expectant audience, frustrated and embarrassed as the conversation stops and your awkward silence continues. It feels as if all the circuitry in your brain has ground to a halt, and if you imagine what's going on inside your head, all you can picture is that interminable Apple rainbow spinning wheel of death.

Eventually, blessedly, the word pops into your consciousness. You remember, and the relief is palpable. But you're left with a lingering stressor, one that feels bigger and carries more foreboding. What was that glitch all about?

Most likely, this episode is an example of normal, no-need-to-see-a-neurologist, middle-aged forgetting. An innocent senior moment. A sign of a memory system getting older and not a sign of disease pathology.

Let's start with the good news. Memory capability doesn't decrease across the board as we age. For example, aging doesn't degrade muscle memory. You won't stop knowing how to ride a bike when you turn fifty, and barring any brain disease or injury, you'll continue to know how to get dressed, feed yourself, use your phone, type e-mails to your grandchildren, and read this book when you're ninety. Muscle memories are stable through the ages. Your *execution* of what you know how to do, however, might not be what it used to be. The muscles of your body might be weaker and less flexible, your reaction time is probably slower, and you can't see and hear as well as you did when you were younger. But you still know how to do what you've learned—if only your aging body were still up to the task.

In general, older adults possess a larger repository of semantic memories (vocabulary and learned information) than younger adults have. With age, we accumulate knowledge, and thankfully, this doesn't go the way of the collagen in your face. Older people know more than younger people do. And we continue to be able to consolidate and store semantic memories as we age. Remember Akira Haraguchi, the retired engineer from Japan who recited pi to 111,700 digits from memory? He was sixty-nine years old when he accomplished this feat. Healthy aging brains continue to be capable of astonishing memory feats.

But as you might have expected, many memory functions

do normally decline as we age. Let's go back to the common cold of forgetting—all those words that go mysteriously missing. *Oh, what's his name?* Normal, age-related forgetting is most pronounced with TOT free recall, and the frequency of TOTs typically upticks around age forty. If you don't have the optimal—or, worse, any—cues, and you're not being asked to recognize a face from a picture or pick the correct word from choices A, B, or C, but you need your brain to simply recall something you know you know, this memory task gets harder as you grow older.

While our free-recall ability might feel as if it's plummeting as we age, recognition and familiarity are thankfully stable. I can't remember the name of the actor who starred in *The Sopranos*, but I'll have no trouble recognizing his name if you show me the answer, even decades from now. Intact recognition also reveals that this semantic information is still safely stored in my brain and that this memory hasn't vanished with age. The missing blocked word is in my head. But the information does become harder to fish out on demand as the years pile up.

Episodic memory recall also decreases normally as we age. We forget more of what happened, but what we can recall is as accurate (and inaccurate) as younger people's recollections. As noted in the discussion on prospective memory in chapter 9, we're all pretty pitiful at reliably remembering what we intend to do later, and after the age of fifty, this less-than-stellar performance only gets worse. Writing down what you need to remember later is not a sign of weakness or cause for shame at any age. It's just good sense.

We also experience a noticeable decline in working memory with age, both in the auditory loop and in the visuospatial scratchpad. So if I rattle off a phone number or a Wi-Fi password, you'll have a harder time holding that information in your working memory when you're sixty than at forty. Information evaporates from your present moment faster as you get older.

Processing speeds normally begin diminishing in our thirties, which means it takes longer to learn new information and longer to retrieve stored information. Your ability to sustain attention also decreases as you age. So you're less able to block out distracting stimuli when you're fifty than when you were thirty, and because you need to pay attention to create new memories, your ability to remember suffers.

Retrieval takes a hit here, too. Decades before my grandmother had any signs of Alzheimer's, she would often call me Anne or Laurel or Mary. She had five daughters and four daughters-in-law and many more granddaughters. As she got older, she was less able to ignore these related, competing, and distracting names when trying to retrieve mine.

You also become less able to attend to more than one thing at a time as you age. And so if two things are going on at once, you are less likely to remember either one of them, much less both. Moreover, new associations between previously unrelated pieces of information are harder to remember as you age.

So you can recall monkey-banana as well as younger people can, but you're less likely to remember monkey-airplane.

Retrieval begins to don rose-colored glasses as we grow older, and we show an increasing tendency to recall the good stuff and forget the bad. For example, younger and older adults shown a series of pictures that were either emotionally positive, neutral, or negative were later tested for recall of the images. As we would expect, older folks remembered fewer pictures overall than did the younger adults. The younger crowd recalled the emotional photos better than they remembered the neutral images, and positive and negative images were remembered equally well. But the older group recalled twice as many positive pictures as negative, and the number of negative photos recalled was about the same as the number of neutral images. When shown the previously forgotten emotionally negative photos, the older people recognized all of them easily. So these photos made it into their memories, but when they were asked to recall what they had seen, these emotionally negative images weren't consciously retrievable.

Surely there must be something we can do to combat aging's normal but corrosive effects on memory performance. These declines in memory creation, retrieval, and processing speed aren't all inevitable, are they? You're not going to like this, but it appears the answer is *ultimately* yes. If you eat a daily diet of doughnuts, only go for a run if someone is chasing you, regularly sacrifice sleep by binge-watching entire seasons of the latest show on Netflix until 3 A.M., and are chronically stressed, you'll most definitely accelerate the aging of your memory. Alternatively, if you eat a Mediterranean or a MIND diet (a combination of the Mediterranean diet and DASH diet, which I'll discuss later in the book), exercise regularly, meditate daily, and sleep for eight hours a night, you'll absolutely improve your memory performance in the near term. You will also probably extend the lifespan of your youthful memory for longer. These healthy lifestyle choices can also potentially prevent dementia. But lifestyle can't bail water out of an old, leaky boat forever.

Think of your skin as an analogy. If you bask in the hot sun without sunscreen every day, your skin will age faster than if you wear a hat and sunscreen and mostly stay indoors. But eventually, no matter what you do, if you live long enough, your skin, like your memory, is going to age. And just as some of us wrinkle and sag more or less than others do, your memory will be affected by age differently from the same-aged person next to you. Some seventy-year-olds have sharper, more responsive recall than do other seventy-year-olds. But for the most part, their memory performance is likely to be slower and less powerful than it was when these same folks were thirty.

What about applying the adage of "use it or lose it" to your aging brain? Can keeping mentally active preserve your memory's performance as you get older? While staying cognitively active is one tool we can use to build an Alzheimer's-resistant brain, there is no compelling data to support that doing so self-testing, creating meaning, using visual and spatial imagery, keeping a diary—will improve memory at any age. They may have a less powerful effect on your memory performance at seventy than they would if you were thirty, but these methods still work. Akira Haraguchi might have been able to memorize pi to 200,000 digits if he had tried when he was twenty-nine, but what his sixty-nine-year-old memory was capable of recalling through repetition, focus, visual imagery, and story is still phenomenally impressive. These tools are available to your memory, too, at any age. You just have to use them.

13

Alzheimer's

"Two weeks ago, I woke up next to my wife of thirty-four years, and it took me ten minutes to figure out who she was. I knew she was someone of interest, but I couldn't connect the dots." This is but one of the countless and devastating memory failures my friend Greg O'Brien has shared with me. An acclaimed journalist, Greg introduced himself to me several years ago in an e-mail. It seemed like a note meant to woo and wow me, and just as I was thinking this, I read:

> Don't be overly impressed by the articulation of this email. It took about two hours to write. Years ago, I

would have written this in five minutes or less. But it was worth the time.

Greg had been diagnosed two years earlier with early-onset Alzheimer's at the age of fifty-nine. People regularly ask me if there is a clear difference between forgetting due to normal aging and forgetting due to Alzheimer's. The answer? Definitely.

That first e-mail from Greg was the beginning of one of my life's greatest friendships. Over the years, as this disease continues to progressively steal his memory, we've talked about pretty much everything—the good, the bad, the ugly, and the really hideous. There was the time he met me at a coffee shop in the middle of winter wearing soaking wet clothes. I hugged him and, feeling the cold damp of his shirt in my hands, asked, "What's going on here?" When he had pulled his clothes out of the dryer at home, they were still wet. Unable to remember how to work the machine or to pivot his thinking to a new plan that would involve retrieving dry clothes from his closet, Greg dressed himself in the wet clothes.

Another time, we were at a book signing together when he leaned over and whispered, "I can't remember how to write the letter *Q*." I drew it on a scrap of paper and passed it to him under the table like a misbehaving kid in class.

Back when he was still driving and I was lovingly pestering

him to give up driving, he unexpectedly saw a deer in the middle of the road, swerved, and flipped his Jeep. As he was upside down, moments before what could have been his death, he said he thought, "Lisa Genova is going to kill me."

So what's going on inside Greg's brain? Memory impairment due to Alzheimer's (often called *dementia,* an umbrella term that includes deficits in memory, language, and cognition) isn't caused by slower processing speeds or diminished attention. In the beginning stages of Alzheimer's, dementia results from a molecular war in the neural synapses involved in consolidating and retrieving memories, rendering those connections impassible. In later stages of the disease, forgetting is caused by the death and loss of the neurons themselves.

Although the molecular causes of Alzheimer's are still debated, most neuroscientists believe the disease begins when a protein called *amyloid beta* starts forming plaques in our synapses. In the earliest part of the disease, the person is blissfully unaware. During this stage, many years ago now, Greg wasn't experiencing any symptoms of abnormal forgetting. We think it takes fifteen to twenty years of seemingly innocent amyloid plaque accumulation before it reaches a tipping point, then triggering a molecular cascade that causes tangles, neuroinflammation, cell death, and pathological forgetting.

Think of amyloid plaques as a lit match. The lit match alone doesn't cause a problem, but at the tipping point, the match sets fire to the forest. Your brain is now ablaze with

Alzheimer's disease. And you are now experiencing significant, abnormal memory loss.

On the bright side, it takes a really long time for our brains to develop Alzheimer's. But here's the bad news—if you're over forty, you're likely to have amyloid plaques accumulating in your brain right now. Before these plaques accumulate to the tipping point, your lapses in memory might look something like this:

> Why did I come into this room?
> Oh, what's his name?
> Where did I put my keys?

Utterly maddening, but 100 percent normal. After the tipping point, the glitches in memory function are markedly different from normal forgetting. Well past the tipping point, Greg regularly forgets what happened a few minutes ago, what he or I just said, and what happened yesterday.

"I wake up in the morning and can't remember what I did," he says. "Happens all the time. Or I'm writing in a coffee shop and someone I know comes over to say hello. We chat. Then an hour later, that person will come over again, and I'll say, 'Great to see you. How are you?' And the person will say, 'We already chatted about an hour ago.' And I have no memory of the conversation or of even seeing that person."

Alzheimer's begins in the hippocampus, which by now you

know is a brain structure essential for the formation of new, consciously held memories. Thus, the first symptom of Alzheimer's is typically forgetting what happened earlier today or even moments ago and why people with Alzheimer's repeat the same story or question over and over. This kind of rapid forgetting isn't normal. Older memories already formed are safe for now, but new information that would normally be consolidated into a lasting memory by the hippocampus and available later for retrieval is lost. People with Alzheimer's can forget what they ate for lunch an hour ago (or even that they had lunch) and still be able to tell you in great detail a story about walking to school sixty years ago.

But we've all experienced forgetting something your spouse just said, losing your train of thought in a conversation, not remembering whether you turned off the oven five minutes ago. How are these everyday lapses different from Alzheimer's? If you don't have Alzheimer's and you pay attention to what your partner is saying, you're going to remember what they said (really, folks, try it). Paying attention to what I'm saying doesn't guarantee a thing for Greg. Making new memories when you have Alzheimer's is hard and only grows harder, because less and less of your hippocampus is available to do the job.

Failure to retrieve the right words is another early symptom of Alzheimer's. But I already told you that *Oh, what's his name?* is normal and typically increases in frequency with age. So the next time you block on the actor who played Tony Soprano, see the person, 70 percent of the time now, he can't come up with this individual's name. Blank.

> I tell the person that I have a memory problem. The person usually responds, "It's OK, Greg," and then tells me their name, usually followed by a hug. Perhaps this is the start of dementia-friendly attitudes. I think the hug is not pity for me but a realization that they could face the same journey someday.

Before he had Alzheimer's, when trying to recall a blocked name or word, Greg used to do what most of us do—search the brain. Go through the letters of the alphabet. Wade through neural circuits in an attempt to hunt down or even stumble across the neural circuit connected to the word. *Hold on. I know it's in there. If I can just activate the right neurons.* With Alzheimer's, Greg knows that the word isn't going to float to the surface on its own, because it's drowning in the murky quagmire of disease.

So, he bypasses his brain and searches Google instead:

> I keep my laptop with me at all times. I play charades with Google—"sounds like," describing in general the name, event, or place. So if I'm trying to remember the word *Broadway*, I'll type "Places in NYC for

> entertainment," see what that pulls up. If I don't find it, I might add "Where the ball drops in NYC on New Year's Eve." I'll get "Times Square" as a result. Then I'll type "Times Square in NYC" or "Best plays in NYC."
>
> Of course, I often go down some rabbit hole here and never find what I was looking for. If I get lost or distracted, I hit the arrow back button over and over to retrace my steps. Sometimes I can figure out what I was looking for that way. Sometimes, it's just gone.

Unfortunately, Alzheimer's doesn't just stay put in the hippocampus. It goes on a murderous road trip, invading other regions of the brain. As it spreads to the parietal lobes, where spatial information is processed, people with Alzheimer's start getting lost in familiar places. If you've read *Still Alice,* you might remember that Alzheimer's was interfering with the retrieval of Alice's spatial memories when she found herself suddenly lost in Harvard Square, a neighborhood she had known as home for twenty-five years. (In the movie, which relocated this story to New York City, Alice became disoriented and lost on Columbia University campus.)

Alzheimer's will also compromise neural circuits in the prefrontal and frontal cortices—the most newly developed parts of the brain. With these regions affected, individuals experience impairments in logical thinking, decision-making, planning, and problem-solving. When Greg couldn't reroute his thinking to a plan that involved wearing dry clothes instead of the wet clothes from the dryer, he was experiencing Alzheimer's in his frontal cortex.

We'll also start seeing memory impairments arising from a compromised ability to pay attention. People with Alzheimer's start misplacing their keys, wallets, phones, glasses, laptops, and money. As a distracted human in today's world, we all regularly experience *Where's my X?* moments. How can we know if these are normal or an early symptom of Alzheimer's?

If you eventually find your keys on the table by the front door or in your coat pocket, your moment of forgetfulness is probably normal. Frustrating, but nothing to worry about. You most likely didn't pay attention to where you put them. Your amyloid plaque levels are still below the tipping point.

If instead, you find your keys in the refrigerator, this episode is more concerning. If you find your keys and think for a moment, *What are these for?*, then you are not experiencing a sign of a normally aging memory. Forgetting what keys are used for is a semantic memory failure that could be a symptom of disease pathology in your memory system.

Earlier I shared a story about not being able to find my car in a parking garage. I had been in a rush and hadn't paid attention to where I parked before I abandoned my car and ran off to speak at a conference. Less than two hours later, I returned to the garage and couldn't remember where I had parked. I paced up and down ramps with no luck. Just as I had concluded that my car must have been stolen, I happened on it. But the culprit behind my missing car wasn't a failure in memory retrieval at all. It was a failure of attention. I hadn't actually forgotten anything. Without giving the parking spot my attention, I never formed a memory of its location in the first place.

Consider Greg's experience. Back when he was still driving, he drove his yellow Jeep to the dump. He got out, dumped his trash, and then he stood there, stumped, wondering how he was going to get home. In the space of a minute, he had forgotten that he had driven there. His yellow Jeep was waiting right in front of him, but this most obvious of all cues couldn't activate either the episodic memory (*You just drove to the dump*) or the semantic memory (*That yellow Jeep right there belongs to you*).

He began problem-solving as best he could and thought about his options. "I could call Connor [his son]. I could walk. I could ask someone here to give me a ride. I looked around for someone to take me home, never remembering that I drove here. Never realizing that I was standing directly in front of my yellow Jeep."

And then, suddenly, somehow, the cue found a neural pathway that wasn't blocked by disease and triggered the activation of these memories. "Wait, that's my Jeep. I drove here. I can drive home. The light flickers off in the brain, and then, thankfully, it flickers back on." For now.

Alzheimer's also gunks up the amygdala and limbic system,

brain regions that control mood and emotion. So grief, rage, and lust might become dysregulated and disinhibited. Your dad, who was always very calm, is now prone to fits of frightening rage. Greg experiences rage regularly. My grandmother began touching every handsome man in the supermarket.

Alzheimer's also invades the circuitry that houses your muscle memories. When this happens, people with Alzheimer's forget how to do the things they learned how to do. Greg forgot how to write the letter *Q*. My grandmother forgot how to manage her checkbook, how to play bridge, and how to cook. Eventually, people with Alzheimer's will forget how to dress, how to toilet themselves, how to eat an ice cream cone, and how to swallow food.

While Alzheimer's first interferes with the formation of new memories, it eventually and in some ways most tragically destroys the networks of neural connections that house our oldest already-stored memories. At this stage, my grandmother no longer knew who I was. I'm dreading the day when Greg no longer remembers me. In the absence of a cure, that day will sadly and surely come.

Progression from the first symptoms of forgetting to end-stage Alzheimer's takes an average of eight to ten years. This disease eventually and profoundly impairs the formation and retrieval of every kind of memory. Forgetting due to Alzheimer's is pervasive, catastrophic, tragic, and not normal.

PART III

Improve or Impair

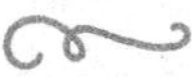

14

Put It in Context

Whether you remember or forget anything is influenced by many factors. As you've already learned, memory creation requires attention. Paying attention is the number one thing you can do to improve your memory at any age, and a lack of attention will impair it. Every time. You've also seen that rehearsal, self-testing, visual and spatial imagery, mnemonics, surprise, emotion, and meaning all improve memory. What else boosts or blocks memory formation and retrieval? Often, our ability to remember depends on the context.

Without my glasses, I can no longer read menus, washing instructions on clothing tags, the labels on medication bottles, or books. The other night as I was settling into bed, excited to snuggle into the next chapter of the book I was reading, I realized that I didn't have my glasses with me. *Sigh. I probably left them in the kitchen.*

I climbed out of bed, padded down the stairs, walked into the kitchen, and flicked on the lights. I looked around, totally stumped. I had no idea why I was in this room.

My brain began playing detective. I knew I had gotten out of bed and come down to the kitchen to get something. But what? I scanned the room—refrigerator, toaster, bananas in a bowl, my jacket hanging on the back of one of the bar stools. Nothing came to mind. Did I come in here to grab something to eat? No. Did I need water? No. I couldn't remember.

Defeated, I returned to my bedroom, and pop! *My glasses!* Back downstairs I went. At least I was getting some exercise.

Forgetting the reason you've walked into a room is one of the most common memory failure complaints I hear, right behind forgetting names and where you put your keys and phone. We all experience walking into a room only to scratch our heads in dumbfounded wonder. Why am I here?

Why does this happen? In my example, I literally had the thought *Go get your glasses in the kitchen* only seconds before I physically arrived there. How did this thought, this memory, evaporate so quickly from my mind? Why did my memory of what I intended to do fail in the kitchen and succeed moments later in the bedroom? Why did I have to think and think to no avail in the kitchen but, in my bedroom, remember what I wanted instantly and without effort?

The answer has to do with context. Memory retrieval is far easier, faster, and more likely to be fully summoned when the context of recall matches the context that was present when the memory was formed. We see this phenomenon with prospective (what you plan to do), episodic (what happened), semantic (information you know), and muscle (how to do things) memories.

In the example I just gave, the memory for what I wanted—go to the kitchen to get your glasses—was encoded in my bedroom, surrounded by a specific context colored with cues: bedtime, the copy of *Untamed* on my nightstand, the books in my bookcases. When I arrived in the kitchen, there was nothing to remind me of what I wanted. The refrigerator, the toaster, the bananas in a bowl, my jacket. There were no cues in the kitchen (other than the glasses, which I didn't notice) to trigger the memory of what I needed. And what's more, these kitchen cues actually misdirected the hunt, sending me down neural pathways associated with breakfast and the unseasonably chilly weather, neural circuits that would *not* lead to reading glasses. The context of the kitchen instead interfered with my ability to remember what I went in there for. As soon as I returned to my bedroom, I was standing amid the cues that were present when I created the intention. Retrieval was now effortless and immediate.

We're all more likely to accurately remember something if learning and recall happen under the same conditions. My favorite study on context- or state-dependent memory involves a bunch of deep-sea divers on and off the coast of Scotland. Half learned a list of unrelated words twenty feet UNDERWATER. The other half learned the same list ON THE BEACH. Later, everyone was asked to write down as many words as they could remember from the list, and they were asked to recall these words either UNDERWATER or ON THE BEACH. Here were the four groups:

Learned the list UNDERWATER and asked to recall the list UNDERWATER

Learned the list UNDERWATER and asked to recall the list ON THE BEACH

Learned the list ON THE BEACH and asked to recall the list ON THE BEACH

Learned the list ON THE BEACH and asked to recall the list UNDERWATER

What happened? Recall was significantly better when the test conditions matched the learning conditions. If divers learned the words underwater, they remembered more words underwater than if tested on the beach. Likewise, if divers learned the words on the beach, they tested better on the beach than underwater. Matching the context you're in for recall with the conditions you were in when you learned the information improves recall. Mismatched conditions impair recall.

Since most of us aren't deep-sea divers, let's think of a more relatable example. Have you ever returned to your elementary school, your childhood home, or your childhood neighborhood, and your consciousness was suddenly flooded with vivid, elaborately detailed memories from that time in your life? Let's say you grew up on a farm in rural Vermont, but now you're a fifty-five-year-old corporate suit working in a thirtieth-floor office in Manhattan. If I asked you to tell me about some memories from when you were ten years old, you would probably have little to offer. Out of context, these memories aren't readily available. But if we were to take a road trip north and visit your hometown, you would probably have lots of stories to share. The picket fence, the weeping willow tree, the street signs, Mrs. Daly's house, the red barn—the context would trigger the retrieval of long-forgotten memories consolidated there, memories you might not have thought about in thirty, forty, fifty years. These memories are context-dependent.

But context means more than just where you were when you formed or recalled a memory. It can also mean whom you were with, the time of day or year, the weather. Nor is it limited to what's outside of you. Context can be internal—your emotional or physiological state.

It's much easier to recall memories that match the mood you're in. You're more likely to remember the good times when you're in a good mood and the miserable times when you're feeling depressed (which might then support and exacerbate your gloomy state). When you're mad at your spouse, you're more likely to remember all the bad things about him. That list is at your fingertips and long. When you're in love, your partner is perfect in every way.

Were you hungry, hot, tired, stressed, or thirsty when you were studying for that exam or preparing for that presentation? You'll be better able to recall that information if you're in the same state as you were when you learned it. Similarly, if you learn something when you're caffeinated, then your memory for what you learned will be best if you're caffeinated when trying to recall it.

Why would this be so? The spreadsheet you're studying isn't the only thing that gets consolidated into memory. Everything you experience while you study those numbers is potentially bound into memory as well. The context—both external and internal—becomes part of the memory, and activation of any part of the memory can serve to trigger retrieval of the other parts.

Let's say you're studying for a vocabulary test. While you're studying, you're also listening to Eminem, smelling a lavender-scented candle, and eating sour gummy bears. Let's also say you're tired because you stayed up until 2 A.M. last night binge-watching several seasons of *Friends* instead of studying your vocab words. And maybe you're anxious because you want to get a good grade but you still don't know the words, and you're feeling nauseated from eating too many sour gummy bears. Your best bet for scoring an A is to take the test while feeling tired, anxious, nauseated, wearing lavender-scented body lotion, snacking on gummy bears, and singing Eminem in your head. You will not want to take that exam well slept, relaxed, eating kale chips, and listening to Mozart.

Even language can provide context. Say your grandmother is Italian and immigrated to the United States when she was twelve years old. She has spoken English since. If you ask her about a childhood memory, she's likely to answer you in Italian (or she might retrieve the memory in her head in Italian and then translate it for you).

So the next time you walk into a room and stop cold because you cannot for the life of you remember why you went in there, don't freak out. This blank state is not an existential crisis or a reason to suspect Alzheimer's. But don't just stand there trying to muscle the answer into your consciousness, either. Your brain doesn't work that way. Go back to the room you were in before walking into this one—either literally or in

15

Stressed Out

Unless you're the Dalai Lama, you're probably consumed by regular if not daily doses of significant stress. A viral pandemic, another mass shooting, more political division, losing your job, college tuition, an astronomical medical bill, deadlines at work, traffic, raising children, divorce, a sick parent, loneliness, uncertainty about the health and longevity of your marriage, your job, the country, our planet. Approximately 79 percent of Americans say they feel stress sometimes or frequently every single day.

Plenty of scientific evidence demonstrates that relentless, unmanaged stress is toxic for your body and brain. Chronic stress can contribute to the development of many diseases and ailments, such as type 2 diabetes, heart disease, cancer, infections, pain disorders, panic attacks, insomnia, depression, and Alzheimer's disease. Lacking effective tools to combat incessant stress, too many people fall victim to addiction and "deaths of despair." Stress itself isn't deadly, but excessive exposure to it creates the opportunity for many other things to kill you.

But what about your memory? Is stress good or bad for memory? Like context, it depends.

Stress is any perceived danger, threat, or challenge. Back in the day, let's say a million years ago, stress was largely external. You noticed that a predator or an enemy was about to attack you, and your brain and body instantly activated the stress response, allowing you to react.

But times have changed dramatically. As you're reading this book right now in modern times, you're presumably and hopefully not in a life-or-death situation. You're probably sitting on a comfy couch. Maybe you've got a soft blanket draped across your lap. Nothing external is physically threatening your well-being.

But the thoughts inside your head can be a dangerous experience. Because we can remember, imagine, ruminate, and worry, we might—internally—be running for our lives. Psychological stress can be caused by a perceived lack of certainty, control, predictability, social support, or belonging. And even if the stressor you're perceiving or anticipating never happens, you will have lived through the stress response in your brain and body by simply imagining it. When it comes to experiencing stress, your thoughts are as real as a hungry lion or an armed gunman in your living room.

This acute stress response is your fight-or-flight, sympathetic nervous system response. When the amygdala senses a challenge or threatening situation, it instantly sends an alarm signal to the hypothalamus. The hypothalamus then passes the baton via a neurotransmitter to the pituitary gland, which then releases a hormone into the bloodstream. The hormone then acts on the adrenal glands, which sit on top of your kidneys, telling them to release stress hormones.

The two workhorse stress hormones released by your adrenal glands are adrenaline and cortisol. *Adrenaline* is a fast-acting, short-lived emergency alarm, mobilizing your brain and body to act right now. It increases your heart rate, respiration, and blood pressure, diverting blood and energy away from everything that isn't essential such as cell growth and digestion (no sense digesting that meal if you might be killed in the next five minutes) and toward your limbs *(Run! Fight!)*. It also enhances your senses and ability to focus while inhibiting your ability to think, so you can respond right away without taking the time to weigh the pros and cons.

Cortisol is a little slower than adrenaline. Whereas adrenaline is on the scene within seconds, cortisol is busiest fifteen minutes to an hour after the onset of the stressor. Cortisol mobilizes glucose (energy) so that you can physically respond to the stressful situation. Importantly, it also shuts off the entire stress response.

This response is meant to be a temporary, quick-on and quick-off physiological state adaptive for survival. It mobilizes the brain and body to react to an immediate threat or challenge. And it isn't bad for you. Quite the contrary, you need this stress response to function normally every day—to give that presentation today at work, to hit the brakes when the car in front of you unexpectedly stops, and even to pry yourself out of bed in the morning.

So how does an acute stressor affect memory? In a nutshell, it helps you form new memories about the stressful situation you're in, but it impairs your ability to retrieve memories already made. But let's crack this nutshell open a bit more, because there are nuances.

Acute stress generally facilitates the formation of new memories. First, a brief burst of something stressful increases your attention, and as you know from earlier in the book, paying attention is essential for the formation of memories. Second, in addition to mobilizing your body and brain for immediate action, adrenaline and cortisol also activate the release of a neurotransmitter called *norepinephrine* in your amygdala. In response, your amygdala sends a signal to your hippocampus, which essentially communicates, "Hey, this stressful thing that's going on right now is probably vitally important—consolidate it! Make a memory!" Cortisol can also act directly on receptors in the hippocampus to promote memory consolidation.

So if we're considering a single, temporarily stressful event, then stress improves memory formation. Giving cortisol to subjects just before they view stressful pictures enhances their memory of these pictures when the subjects are tested later. Without your adrenal glands, you would have a weaker memory for information and events that occur while you're stressed than do people with adrenal glands.

But while exposure to acute stress enhances the formation of new memories, it doesn't boost your ability to remember *everything.* Because our senses and attention become heightened but narrowed during the fight-or-flight response, the menu of details available for consolidation into memory is also narrowed. So we show an enhanced memory for information central to the stressful situation but worse memory for details in the periphery. For example, if you were to witness an armed bank robbery (pretty stressful), you're likely to remember vivid details about the gun (the central source of your stress) but maybe not the number of people in the bank or what the bank tellers looked like.

Additionally, while acute stress improves memory formation for the central details of the stressful experience, it does not facilitate memory formation for neutral information. Subjects injected with adrenaline and shown neutral pictures showed no better memory formation than did saline-injected control subjects. And stress doesn't enhance the formation of memories unrelated to the stressor. Say you're a college student studying for a physics exam you have in the morning. You've got a lot of complex information to master, you're under time pressure, and you want to get an A. All this acute stress will help you consolidate the information you're trying to learn. But if your roommate interrupts your studying to share a story about the time she traveled to Iceland, your elevated stress level won't improve your ability to form a memory for the story just told. Your roomie's story about Iceland is unrelated to the stress you're feeling about your physics exam.

The degree of acute stress you're experiencing also matters. If we were to plot the relationship between perceived stress and memory formation, the graph would take the shape of an inverted *U*. Too little stress about the physics exam, and you won't have enough activation of your amygdala to enhance memory consolidation in your hippocampus. Too much stress, and you're in an overwhelmed state, unable to pay attention to, or process, much of anything. There's an optimal level of temporary stress for creating memories related to the stressful situation, and this level differs by the individual. Some of us have a great deal of tolerance for acute stress, whereas others crack under pressure.

While being temporarily stressed out can facilitate the formation of new memories, stress can also impair your ability to retrieve memories that are already stored. Imagine you've studied for a final exam. You know the information cold. You're confident and ready to ace the test. But when you reach the classroom, you suddenly feel anxious. Your heart is pounding, your hands are sweaty, and your stomach is in knots. You read the first question and draw a total blank. You know you know the answer, but your brain can't retrieve it. And being stumped only adds to the stress you're experiencing.

Many studies demonstrate that stress jams up memory retrieval. For example, subjects given cortisol show deficits in fetching previously learned information compared with subjects given saline. If the release of cortisol is blocked, retrieval of established memories is normal.

So temporary, moderate stress improves memory formation, though it can impair recall. But what happens if you're regularly or constantly stressed out, as most of us are? Is chronic stress ever good for your memory? No. In fact, unrelenting stress is disastrous for your memory.

Here's what happens. Let's say whatever is stressing you out doesn't go away—you have a tyrannical boss, an abusive partner, a sick child. Or you're hit with stressor after stressor after stressor—you were in a car accident and you broke your arm and then you lost your job and now you can't pay your bills. Your fight-or-flight response is being hammered over and over, and cortisol is released every time. The shutoff valve in your hypothalamus soon becomes desensitized to the presence of so much cortisol and stops responding. As a result, the stress response stays turned on. Your brain and body are now in a sustained runaway-train state of fight or flight.

This does not help your memory. When chronic stress continually alerts your amygdala, you'll be spending too much time and energy in your primitive, emotional brain and not in your thinking brain. Stress inhibits your prefrontal cortex, impairing your ability to think. You can react immediately, without taking the time to consider the pros and cons of doing this or that, which is great if you have to run away from a lion right now. But under chronic stress, you're going to have a hard time thinking clearly.

Even more concerning, if you're under constant stress, you'll start losing neurons in your hippocampus. You might have heard somewhere along the way that if you kill off an adult neuron, it's gone for good—that adult brain cells can't regenerate. This dogma was debunked in the 1990s. Neurogenesis (the growth of new neurons) occurs throughout life in many parts of your brain and most notably in your hippocampus . . . unless your hippocampus is constantly soaking in a cortisol bath. Chronic stress inhibits neurogenesis in the hippocampus. So if you're experiencing unrelenting, unmanaged stress, you'll have a smaller hippocampus, which means fewer neurons available to consolidate memories, which means your ability to create new memories will be impaired.

Hippocampal neurons under continual exposure to stress and cortisol also seem to be more vulnerable to damage by other insults, such as a stroke or Alzheimer's disease. In a study of perceived stress levels in eleven hundred women aged thirty-eight to sixty over thirty-five years, women who reported experiencing chronic stress had a 65 percent increased risk of Alzheimer's. In another study, people under chronic stress were twice as likely to develop Alzheimer's disease as were people who felt less stress, and the chronically stressed people were ten times more likely to develop cognitive impairment over five years.

So chronic stress is bad for your memory. But life today is stressful. We can't control world politics or the weather or the next pandemic. You can't get rid of your hostile boss, an overwhelming deadline, or the seemingly endless traffic jam you're sitting in. You can't prevent stress from walking through your front door all day long. So what can we do? Are we doomed to live in a constant sweaty-palmed state of anxiety with shrunken hippocampi stewing in a soup of ineffective cortisol, unable to remember what we just read because we're so stressed out?

While we can't necessarily free ourselves from the stress in our lives, we can dramatically influence our brain's and body's response to each stressful situation we find ourselves in. Through yoga, meditation, a healthy diet, exercise, and practices in mindfulness, gratitude, and compassion, we can train ourselves to become less reactive, to put the brakes on the runaway stress response, to stay healthy in the face of toxic anxiety. All of these approaches have been shown to reduce chronically elevated blood pressure, inflammation, anxiety, and perceived stress. They also restore cortisol levels. These chronic-stress busters may also improve your memory by enhancing neurogenesis in the hippocampus. For example, the hippocampi in the brains of people who meditated for thirty minutes a day were significantly bigger after eight weeks than this region was before the people began this daily practice. Age-matched folks who didn't meditate showed no change in the size of their hippocampi. Similar results have been found in those who regularly exercise.

In considering the long list of stressors you encounter regularly, I would bet that forgetting is one of them. Do you become frustrated, fearful, or worried every time you can't remember a name, forget to pick up your dry cleaning, or puzzle over where you put your phone? Are you frequently stressed out about these kinds of routine lapses in memory?

Now that you understand that acute stress can interfere with recall and that chronic stress can literally shrink your hippocampus, you know that fretting about forgetting can be a self-fulfilling prophecy. So let's all take a collective deep breath. The next time you struggle with the name of that famous surfer or forget to buy milk at the store, you can remember that these are examples of normal forgetting and, hopefully, you can relax. Forgetting happens. If you stress about it, it will happen even more.

16

Go to Sleep

If big pharma came out with a pill tomorrow that could improve your memory and significantly lower your risk of Alzheimer's, would you take it? How much would you pay for that medication? Well, we already have it.

It's called sleep.

When I was a kid, my friends and I sometimes fantasized about being superheroes. Powers regularly on our wish lists were flying, invisibility, and time travel. I was down with all those, but I also always dreamed of possessing the superpower of never needing to sleep.

I still wish for this power. Imagine all the books I could

read and write, the languages I could learn, everything I could accomplish if only I didn't need to waste all those hours being unconscious!

Assuming a nightly slumber of eight hours (fully realizing that few of us regularly get this much), we humans spend a third of our lives asleep. If you're lucky enough to live to the age of eighty-five, then you'll have spent 248,200 hours asleep. That's the equivalent of twenty-eight full years sleeping! If you're fifty, that means you've already spent sixteen years of your life asleep. That's sixteen years of not reading, not working, not thinking, not socializing, not playing, and not loving. Similarly, other animals aren't hunting, eating, mating, or grooming while sleeping, either. Why would humans and other animals have evolved to devote so much time to doing nothing?

The answer lies in the question. Sleep is not an optional state of doing nothing. It's not a passive, blank slate state of unconsciousness, a pathetic period of rest for the unmotivated, an unfortunate waste of time, or even simply the absence of wakefulness. Sleep is a biologically busy state that is vital to your health, your survival, and your optimal functioning. Insufficient sleep puts you at a higher risk for heart disease, cancer, infection, mental illness, Alzheimer's, and memory impairment.

Sleep is clearly doing something superpowerful.

With respect to memory, sleep plays a critical role in many

ways. First, you need sleep to pay attention. If you don't get enough sleep tonight, your frontal cortex is going to be dragging itself to its desk job in the morning, and your ability to concentrate is going to be sluggish. You know now that the first step in creating a memory is noticing what you're going to remember. And to notice anything, you need to both perceive it and pay attention to it. So by ensuring that your frontal cortex neurons are alert, active, and ready for duty, sleep provides you with the attention you need to encode new memories.

But attention-boosting is probably the least impressive of sleep's powerful effects on memory. Sleeping also hits the SAVE button on these newly encoded memories. It saves memories in two steps: First, the unique pattern of neural activity that occurred in your brain when you were experiencing, learning, and even rehearsing something while awake is reactivated during sleep. This neural replay is thought to facilitate the linking of these connections, cementing them into a single memory. In fact, the amount of replay that occurs during the consolidation process while you snooze correlates with the amount of memory you'll be able to recall after you wake up.

Sleep helps consolidate new memories, and insufficient sleep interferes with consolidation. After a miserable night's sleep, you'll probably go through the next day experiencing a form of retrograde amnesia. Some of your memories from yesterday might be fuzzy, inaccurate, or even missing. Recall for lists, paired associations, patterns, textbook information, and what happened today has been shown to be enhanced by 20 to 40 percent after sleep compared with recall after an equivalent amount of time spent awake. Tomorrow's recall for semantic and episodic memories made today will be significantly better after a night's sleep. This benefit derives from time spent asleep and not just from the passage of time.

In addition to improving episodic and semantic memories, sleep also optimizes muscle memory. We all know that repetition improves skill learning. Practice makes perfect. But what happens if we add sleep to this recipe?

In a study examining the effect of sleep on learning a muscle memory task, subjects were asked to press four numerical keys on the computer in this specific order, 4-1-3-2-4, with their nondominant hand as fast and as accurately as they could for thirty seconds. They practiced this task twelve times, and on average, everyone's performance improved by about 4 percent.

All subjects were tested again on the same task twelve hours later. Half spent those twelve hours awake and demonstrated no improvement in their speed and accuracy. The other half was also tested twelve hours later, but the twelve-hour stretch included a full eight-hour night of sleep. The participants' speed increased by 20 percent, and their accuracy improved by 35 percent. This substantial boost in skill memory was achieved not through continued practice or the simple passage of time. These people improved because they slept!

Sleep appears to be helpful for all muscle memory skills. People need sleep to consolidate the consciously deliberate, separate steps of a task into an automated, seamless muscle memory. Sleeping facilitates skill mastery—when you no longer have to think about the placement of each finger on the piano keys while reading every note on the sheet music and can just play the piece from memory. Without any additional practice, you will be better at what you're learning to do after you've slept. Practice does make perfect, if you sleep on it.

There is also power in napping. The same sequential 4-1-3-2-4 finger-tapping task was used again to see if napping would improve motor memory as much as a full night of slumber would. After learning the task, half of the subjects took a sixty- to ninety-minute nap. The other half stayed awake. The subjects who napped improved their pre-nap performance by 16 percent. The subjects who didn't nap showed no change in performance.

All subjects were tested again the next day, after everyone had enjoyed a full night's sleep. The group that had napped the day before improved their performance further from 16 percent to 23 percent. The group that hadn't napped improved their finger-tapping performance from no improvement to 24 percent. They had caught up with the nappers. So napping can give you an edge in performance that same day, but it doesn't beat what will be gained from a full night's sleep.

Many studies show that people become increasingly worse at learning new things as the day wears on. Unless they nap. But how does a nap improve your ability to remember new things? We're not sure, but here's the hypothesis that most experts are running with. Unlike your cortex, your hippocampus doesn't have infinite storage capacity. Say you're cramming for an exam tomorrow, and you're trying to memorize massive amounts of information. Hypothetically, you can max out your hippocampus. So consolidating even a few of your newly made memories during a nap might free up some much-needed space for consolidating new stuff.

Naps therefore help you retain what you have already learned, and they seem to help make room for what you're going to learn. How long do these naps need to be? A twenty-minute nap should be enough time to give you plenty of memory-boosting benefits without risking the grogginess of sleep inertia that often follows lengthier midday slumbers.

Once a pooh-pooher of naps, author Daniel Pink now swears by them. He also adds an interesting embellishment—the "nappuccino." He drinks coffee just before he nods off for a twenty-minute nap. When he wakes up, many of his newly formed memories will have been consolidated into long-term, stable storage; his maxed-out hippocampus will have been somewhat cleared out, making room for whatever he needs to remember next; and the caffeine from his coffee, which takes about twenty-five minutes to enter his bloodstream, will almost have kicked in, activating his frontal cortex neurons to pay attention. Now that's a power nap.

If I haven't yet convinced you that getting enough sleep is a superpower essential for your memory, buckle your seatbelt. A growing body of evidence suggests that sleep is critical for reducing your risk of Alzheimer's disease. As discussed, most neuroscientists believe that Alzheimer's is caused by an accumulation of amyloid plaques. Normally, amyloid is cleared away and metabolized by glial cells, the janitors of your brain. As a group, these cells form your brain's sewage and sanitation department. During deep sleep, your glial cells flush away any metabolic debris that has accumulated in your synapses while you were in the business of being awake. Deep sleep is like a power cleanse for your brain. And one of the most important things that is cleared away during your nightly slumber is amyloid.

But what happens if you shortchange yourself on deep sleep? The glial cells won't have enough time to finish cleaning your brain, and you will wake up in the morning with amyloid left over in your synapses from yesterday. An amyloid hangover.

A single night of sleep deprivation can lead to an increase in amyloid and tau (another predictive biomarker for Alzheimer's) in cerebral spinal fluid. If you continue to get insufficient sleep, amyloid will continue to accumulate night after night, and you will be closer and closer to the dreaded tipping point—closer and closer to a diagnosis of Alzheimer's.

And amyloid accumulation has been shown to disrupt sleep, which will in turn cause more amyloid to accumulate, and now you're stuck in a dizzying feedback loop that accelerates plaque formation. What does all this information suggest? Insufficient sleep is likely to be a significant risk factor in the development of Alzheimer's.

But how much sleep is enough? Human adults have evolved to require seven to nine hours of sleep per night. Less than that compromises the functioning of your cardiovascular system, immune system, mental health, and memory. Let me repeat this point, because many of you probably just breezed past those words or assumed that five or six hours a night is close enough, or you just didn't believe me. Sleep science data is very clear on this connection between sleep and health. Every night, your sleep processes actively fight off heart disease, cancer, infection, and mental illness. The vitality of every organ system in your body—including your brain—is improved when you get enough sleep, but your health and ability to remember is drastically compromised when you don't. Sleeping less than seven to nine hours a night poses a real risk to your health, both the next day and over a lifetime. Sleep is a mighty superpower, but it wields a double-edged sword.

We used to do a pretty good job of sleeping enough. According to a 1942 Gallup poll, U.S. adults were getting an average of 7.9 hours of sleep per night. But times have changed. Most cultures today have developed a dangerously dismissive attitude toward sleep. In this modern era of relentless busyness, of pressures to have it all and do it all, of skyrocketing anxiety and screen time and late-night hours spent binge-watching the entire second season of *The Marvelous Mrs. Maisel* in one sitting, we are sleeping significantly less than we used to. Today, adults in the United States, the United Kingdom, and Japan sleep an average of about 6.5 hours per night.

We're sleep-deprived, and we tend to be proud of this. But touting a lifestyle of anything less than seven hours of sleep per night is misinformed braggadocio. Sleep experts are unanimous on the amount of nightly slumber we need. We need seven to nine hours a night. Anything less is detrimental to our health and our memories.

In summary, if you don't get seven to nine hours of sleep tonight,

- Your frontal cortex neurons will be sluggish tomorrow, hampering your ability to pay attention and therefore to encode important new memories;
- You won't as clearly and completely remember what you learned and experienced yesterday;

17

Alzheimer's Prevention

Age is the number one risk factor for Alzheimer's. Memory loss due to Alzheimer's is rare under the age of sixty-five, but after that, the numbers change quickly. In the United States, one in ten people at age sixty-five has Alzheimer's. At eighty-five, it's one in three, fast approaching one in two. Half of us.

But we can't do anything about getting older. If we live long enough, is forgetting due to Alzheimer's our brain's destiny? For most of us, it is not. Alzheimer's is not a part of normal aging. Only 2 percent of people with Alzheimer's have the purely inherited, early-onset form of the disease. Ninety-eight percent of the time, Alzheimer's is caused by a combination of the genes we inherited and how we live. While we can't do anything about our DNA, science clearly shows that the way we live can dramatically affect the accumulation of amyloid plaques. This in turn means that, like cancer and heart disease, there are things we can do to prevent Alzheimer's. And since we don't develop Alzheimer's overnight—it can take fifteen to twenty years of amyloid plaque accumulation before we become symptomatic for Alzheimer's—we have plenty of time to implement some strategies for prevention.

Let's start with what you eat and drink. Several studies have now clearly demonstrated that people who eat foods from the Mediterranean diet or the MIND diet (a combination of the Mediterranean diet and DASH [dietary approaches to stop hypertension]) cut their risk of Alzheimer's disease by anywhere from a third to a half. Those results are significant. If I told you that the U.S. Food and Drug Administration just approved a medication that reduces your risk of Alzheimer's by 50 percent, would you take it? You bet you would. Both the Mediterranean and the MIND diets include green leafy vegetables, brightly colored berries, nuts, olive oil, whole grains, beans, and fish (especially fish rich in omega-3 fatty acids, which our bodies don't make on their own).

For years, people have been asking me with a cajoling wink and nod if they should be drinking red wine to prevent Alzheimer's. I disappoint them every time. The answer is no.

There simply is no compelling data to support the contention that red wine reduces your risk of Alzheimer's or other dementias. All the studies that suggested otherwise are too flawed to produce any useful conclusions. Unfortunately, these studies have nonetheless produced misleading headlines and the goblet-clutching urban myth that drinking two glasses of red wine a day is prescriptive for preventing Alzheimer's. But there is zero scientific evidence to support this argument.

Even if the research on resveratrol (the compound in red wine that has been touted as protective to your memory) and brain function in mice revealed amyloid clearance and cognitive improvement (they do not), you would have to drink about twenty glasses of red wine per day to experience an equivalent dosage of resveratrol. To be clear, no studies have demonstrated that drinking any amount of red wine reduces your risk of Alzheimer's. On the flip side, drinking alcohol of any kind is likely to increase your risk of Alzheimer's by interfering with the quality and quantity of your sleep.

What about chocolate? Chocolate has been shown to improve attention (via caffeine), and I've already described how attention is an essential ingredient for memory formation. So that's a plus. But as of now, there is no compelling evidence that shows that chocolate reduces your risk of Alzheimer's. Sorry, folks. Like the research on red wine, the studies on chocolate and Alzheimer's to date have been too poorly designed to produce any useful conclusions. That said, chocolate (especially the dark kind) is a source of antioxidants, which are hypothesized to play a role in reducing the inflammation that contributes to cell death in Alzheimer's. So, in theory, chocolate, like any other food or spice with antioxidant properties, may protect your brain from some of the damage caused by free radicals and inflammation. But we don't yet have this data.

What about coffee? In one longitudinal epidemiological study (a longitudinal study follows the same participants over time), drinking three to five cups of coffee per day at midlife was associated with a 65 percent decreased risk of Alzheimer's. We don't know if this effect is the result of caffeine, antioxidants, an impact on insulin sensitivity, a change in the blood-brain barrier, or something else. Nor do we know if tea offers the same benefit. So we need more studies to further our understanding, but as of now, you can add coffee to your Alzheimer's prevention kit. Still, be mindful of when you drink your last latte of the day. You don't want to offset any potential benefits from the coffee by losing sleep tonight.

People with low vitamin D are twice as likely to develop Alzheimer's as are folks with normal vitamin D levels. So if you're low on this vitamin, take a supplement and get some sunshine. A B_{12} deficiency can cause dementia symptoms that look a lot like Alzheimer's, but these memory impairments are in fact not Alzheimer's in origin. The good news here—your symptoms will resolve with B_{12} supplements or shots. Despite widespread rumors, coconut oil has not been shown to have any effect on forgetting due to Alzheimer's. Likewise, ginkgo biloba does not reduce your risk of dementia.

As a rule of thumb, anything that is good for your heart is good for your brain—and for preventing Alzheimer's. So if you're already mindful of your heart health, this is good news for your brain. High blood pressure, obesity, diabetes, smoking, and high cholesterol all increase your risk of developing Alzheimer's. Some autopsy studies show that as many as 80 percent of people with Alzheimer's disease also had cardiovascular disease. Having increased high-density lipoprotein (HDL, the "good" cholesterol) is associated with a 60 percent decreased risk of Alzheimer's compared with people with low HDL. Statins have been shown to delay the onset of Alzheimer's in people seventy-five or older.

You have already learned about sleep's potential impact on the development of Alzheimer's, but sleep's effects are worth reemphasizing here. Chronic sleep deprivation is a significant risk factor for Alzheimer's. I find this conclusion both terrifying (because of the decades I've already spent staying up too late, getting up too early, and feeding babies throughout the night) and encouraging—because I can do something about it now. If you don't yet have Alzheimer's, that means that your amyloid plaque levels haven't reached the tipping point. However sleep-deprived you've already been in your life is water under the bridge. You can still fight against the daily accumulation of amyloid in your brain by getting enough sleep tonight.

If you do nothing else to lower your risk of Alzheimer's, exercise. Aerobic exercise has been associated with a significantly reduced risk of dementia in many human studies, and it decreases amyloid levels in animal models of the disease. Exercise improves sleep (it decreases the time it takes to fall asleep, increases the quality of sleep, and decreases the number of times you wake up in the night). And as described earlier, sleep improves normal memory and reduces your risk of Alzheimer's. Even a daily brisk walk has been correlated with a 40 percent decreased risk of Alzheimer's. That's not a small impact. Exercise works.

Both physical exercise and mental engagement have been shown to stimulate the growth of new neurons in the hippocampus, which, as described earlier, is essential for memory formation and is the first brain region under attack by Alzheimer's. Exercise and mental stimulation might be a way to fight back and replace neurons that have fallen victim to the disease. Conversely, extended sitting and a lack of cognitive activity have been correlated with brain shrinkage. Older adults with a single copy of *APOE4,* a gene variant associated with an increased risk of Alzheimer's, had a 3 percent decrease in hippocampus size over 1.5 years—but only if they were sedentary. If they exercised, they showed no hippocampal shrinkage. The more you sit, the smaller your hippocampus. Smaller brains tend not to remember as well as bigger brains do.

Finally, if you want to prevent memory loss due to Alzheimer's, learn new things. The symptoms of Alzheimer's are ultimately caused by the loss of synapses. An average brain has over a hundred trillion synapses, which is fantastic news because we have a lot to work with. And this isn't a static number. We gain and lose synapses all the time through neural plasticity. Every time we learn something new, we're creating and strengthening new neural connections, new synapses.

So how can learning new things help us when it comes to Alzheimer's? In the Nun Study, 678 nuns, all of them older than seventy-five when the study began, were followed for more than two decades. They were regularly given physical checkups and cognitive tests, and when they died, their brains were all donated for autopsy. In some of these brains, scientists discovered something surprising. Despite the presence of plaques and tangles and brain shrinkage, what appeared to be unquestionable Alzheimer's, the nuns who had belonged to these brains had shown no behavioral signs of having Alzheimer's disease while they were alive.

How could this be? We think these nuns showed no signs of dementia because they had a high degree of cognitive reserve, that is, they had more functional synapses. People who have more years of formal education, who have greater literacy, and who engage regularly in socially and mentally stimulating activities have more cognitive reserve. They have an abundance and a redundancy of neural connections. So even if Alzheimer's does compromise some synapses, they have many backup, alternate connections, which buffer them from noticing that anything is amiss. These folks have a reduced risk of being diagnosed with Alzheimer's.

So we can be resilient to the presence of Alzheimer's pathology through the recruitment of yet-undamaged pathways. And we create these pathways, this cognitive reserve, by learning new things. Ideally, we want these new things to be as rich in meaning as possible, recruiting sight and sound and associations and emotion.

Building up a cognitive reserve doesn't mean doing crossword puzzles. There is no compelling evidence that doing puzzles or brain-training exercises does anything to decrease your risk of Alzheimer's. You'll improve at doing crosswords, but you're not building a bigger, Alzheimer's-resistant brain. You don't want to simply retrieve information you've already learned, because this type of mental exercise is like traveling down old, familiar streets, cruising neighborhoods you already know.

You want to pave new neural roads. Building an Alzheimer's-resistant brain through cognitive stimulation means learning to play piano, meeting new friends, traveling to a new city, or reading this book. You're welcome.

And if, despite all this, you are someday diagnosed with Alzheimer's, there are three lessons I've learned from my grandmother and Greg and the dozens of other people I've come to know living with this disease:

- Diagnosis doesn't mean you're dying tomorrow. Keep living.
- You won't lose your emotional memory. You'll still be capable of understanding love and joy. You might not remember what I said five minutes ago or even who I am, but you'll remember how I made you feel.
- You are more than what you can remember.

18

The Memory Paradox

People do not consist of memory alone. They have feelings, will, sensibility, moral being. It is here you may touch them and see profound change.

—ALEXANDER LURIA

Memory is essential for the functioning of almost everything you do. Because of memory, you know how to walk, talk, brush your teeth, read these words, and type e-mails. You know where you live, your computer password, and how to calculate a 20 percent tip in your head. You recognize the people you love. Without question, memory is an astounding superpower. But remember, memory can also be that flaky friend who never shows up for your coffee date or that wide-eyed preschooler at Disney World willing to believe anything. Memory, especially for what happened last year or what you intend to do later today, is notoriously incomplete, inaccurate, confabulated, and fallible, its performance often better if externalized, outsourced to Google or your calendar.

So where does that leave us with respect to our relationship with memory? How should we hold it? Do we revere our memory as an omnipotent monarch, or do we throw rotten tomatoes at it, denigrating it (and by extension, ourselves) for its inconvenient shortcomings and foolish mistakes? The most sensible answer lies somewhere in between.

Try bearing the tension of this paradox: Memory is everything and nothing. If that statement feels too extreme, try on this gentler version: Memory is a really big deal, and it's not such a big deal. Maybe we can take it seriously but hold it lightly.

If you consider memory a really big deal, you will value the true awesomeness of your memory enough to take care of it. You'll know that by using the right tools, your memory is unlimited in its potential. You can learn a new language, play a guitar, and score an A on that test. You'll also appreciate your memory, and plenty of research has shown that gratitude is associated with greater happiness and well-being.

At the same time, if you also hold memory as not a big deal, then you'll be comfortable with, and forgiving of, your memory's many imperfections:

You can't remember the name of your third-grade teacher. That's OK. Third grade was a long time ago. Memories left alone fade over time.

You can't remember what you had for dinner last Wednesday. Doesn't matter. It was probably spaghetti.

You forgot to return your child's overdue library book. That happens, especially since the task wasn't scheduled in your calendar.

You can't remember the name of that movie with Sandra Bullock and the football player. Oh well, it will come to you later. Or you can google it right now and be done with it.

Your spouse insists that you left your family vacation at the cottage in Maine three days early two years ago because it rained every day. You remember it being sunny all week, and you left only one day early because your son sprained his ankle and you wanted his doctor to look at it before soccer started. Who's right? Who knows? Who cares? You're probably both wrong. Let it go.

You can't remember whether ONE CENT is on the head or the tail of a penny. Not to worry. You've never

> paid attention to that detail, and knowing it never mattered.

By not engaging in blame or a battle with your memory when it forgets, as it inevitably will, you'll feel calmer and less stressed. And less chronic stress is good for your memory and, like gratitude, your overall well-being.

Some people out there can memorize boggling quantities of information. World record holder Akira Haraguchi recited 111,700 digits of pi from memory. Cellist Yo-Yo Ma has committed tens of thousands of notes to muscle memory. While possessing a highly trained memory surely comes with advantages, it doesn't guarantee superior memory capabilities across the board. Haraguchi forgot his wife's birthday. Yo-Yo Ma forgot his cello in the trunk of a taxi. Nor is a well-trained memory a panacea. Folks with excellent memories aren't immune to experiences of loss, disappointment, and failure. Having a remarkable memory doesn't guarantee happiness or success.

While the ability to memorize a slew of information is impressive and useful, most people would say that remembering the details of what happened in your life is more important. But it can't be that important, because unless you're one of the few people on the planet with highly superior autobiographical memory, you don't actually remember most of it. Our brains aren't designed to retain what is routine or predictable, and most of our lives are spent doing routine, predictable things.

Should remembering more and forgetting less even be a desirable goal? Would your life truly be improved if you could remember the details of every morning shower?

Perhaps a more reasonable expectation of memory is for it to forget everything except what is meaningful. That is, the ability to remember the *meaningful* details of your life is what's important. These are the memories that provide you with a sense of self, a life narrative, and the potential for growth and connection with others. Our brains don't remember everything, but maybe what they remember is enough.

And yet even when the meaningful is forgotten, memory doesn't define what it means to be human. My friend Greg O'Brien has been living with Alzheimer's for the past eleven years. This disease has already robbed him of too many precious long-term memories. More loss will follow. Recent memories are nothing but ghosts and shadows. If memory were everything without also being nothing, then Greg would be utterly devastated. His memory losses are real and frustrating, infuriating, scary, and heartbreaking. But they are not everything. This disease hasn't and won't steal Greg's sense of humor, which he masterfully wields in every interaction I have with him. It hasn't taken away his faith or his ability to be present or to have rich relationships with other people. Greg's memory sucks, and he's one of my best friends. He has a family he loves and who love him, and he's still living a memorable life that matters.

Nor is memory required for feeling the full range of human emotions. You don't need memory to love and feel loved. My grandmother knew none of us when she died of Alzheimer's. She had forgotten her married name, all her grandchildren, and all nine of her kids. She no longer recognized her house as her home or her face in the mirror. She thought that her daughter Mary, who had become her full-time caregiver for the past four years, was a homeless woman whom she had kindly taken in. I wouldn't have traded a cup of coffee for her memory when my nana was in the final years of this disease. But even on the day she died, she knew she was loved. She didn't know who we were, but she loved us back.

Take it seriously. Hold it lightly. Memory isn't everything.

Appendix

What to Do About It All

Knowing what we now know about both the aptitude and the fallibility of memory, it's likely that you don't remember everything you've read in this book. So let's go over the major take-home messages. Our memories for what happened are seldom entirely accurate to begin with and often become even less accurate with recall and reconsolidation. Forgetting what isn't needed is actually quite useful. Our memories diminish with time and age, and this is perfectly normal and not reflective of some disease process. Nevertheless, because we now understand how memory works, there are things we can do to improve it.

If you want to enhance your ability to remember what

happened last week and last year, your new Netflix password, your grocery list, why you came into this room, that guy's name, and where you parked your car, what can you do? What's the best way to get the information you want to remember into your head, and then, once it's in there, how can you most easily and reliably access it on demand? How can you make what you've managed to learn and remember more resistant to forgetting?

1. PAY ATTENTION. You can't remember a thing unless you first give that thing your attention. Decrease distractions (put down your phone). Stop multitasking. Pay active attention to what you hope to remember. Be present to the sensory, emotional, and factual information in front of you. Yoga and mindfulness meditation can help strengthen your ability to sustain attention in the present moment. When you maximize attention, you maximize your ability to remember.

2. SEE IT. Adding a mental picture of what you want to remember enhances memory. Always. In visualizing what you're trying to remember, you're adding more neural connections to it. You're deepening the associations, making the formation of that memory more robust. And so you'll better remember it later.

If you're writing down something that you want to remember, write it in ALL CAPS or highlight it in pink marker or circle it. Add a chart, or doodle a picture. Make what you're trying to remember something you can easily see in your mind's eye.

3. MAKE IT MEANINGFUL. We remember what is meaningful. Full stop. Remember the seasoned London taxi drivers who recalled more street names than the newbie drivers but only if the streets were listed in an order that could be driven? Or the chess masters who could remember the arrangement of more chess pieces on the board but only if the pieces had been placed in playable positions and not randomly? When it comes to memory, meaning is king.

Relate what you're trying to remember to stuff you care about. Create a story about the information or event you're trying to remember. Stories are memorable because they mean something.

4. USE YOUR IMAGINATION. People with the best memories have the best imaginations. To help make a memory unforgettable, use creative visual imagery. Visualize, but go beyond the obvious. Attach bizarre, surprising, disgusting, sexy, vivid, funny, physically impossible, interactive elements to what you're trying to remember, and it will stick. If I need to remember to pick up chocolate milk at the grocery store, I can imagine Dwayne "The Rock" Johnson milking a chocolate-brown cow and Tina Fey lying beneath the udder with her mouth open, chocolate milk splattering all over her face. Make the image as wild and unique as possible, and you'll be much more likely to remember it.

5. **LOCATION, LOCATION, LOCATION.** Even better, put this weird image in a location in your mind's eye. Your brain is wired to remember where things are located in space. Placing that chocolate-brown cow in the middle of my living room instead of nowhere in particular will help me remember the image—and to buy chocolate milk—when I'm at the store, and even more so if my living room is a stop on the guided tour of my memory palace.

Visual and spatial imagery are the special-sauce ingredients in the techniques that author and memory champion Joshua Foer uses to memorize absurdly long strings of numbers and a deck of fifty-two cards in a hundred seconds. Foer says that he also uses wildly weird images perched in specific locations (such as Cookie Monster atop a talking horse inside your front door) to assist him in memorizing speeches, people's names, credit card numbers, and items on a grocery list. He does admit, however, that these techniques require a *lot* of training and are not a memory panacea. You have to remember to take a moment to attach a special image to what you want to remember, and doing so in real time takes effort and creative energy.

In the constantly moving moments of a real day, these techniques probably aren't a conveniently accessible tool for most of us. And just because Foer can memorize the order of fifty-two cards faster than I could probably deal the deck, this talent doesn't guarantee that he can remember what he's looking for when he's standing in front of an open refrigerator door or where he put his phone. And even master rememberer Haraguchi forgot his wife's birthday. So there you go. Memory techniques that rely on visual and spatial imagery don't generalize to enhancing memory across the board—like muscle memory for learning how to ski, or recalling the details of the movie you watched on a plane last month, or remembering a loved one's birthday.

6. MAKE IT ABOUT YOU. I rarely endorse self-centeredness, but I make an exception when it comes to enhancing your memory. Called the *superiority illusion*, the idea goes like this: You are more likely to remember a detail about yourself or something that you did than you are to retain a detail about someone else or something someone else did. Which is easier to remember—the last time you cleaned the kitchen or the last time your spouse or roommate did? Hmm. It could be that this other person never cleans the kitchen, or maybe you're suffering from the superiority illusion.

You can harness your memory's proclivity for self-involvement to better remember other things. Make what you're learning personal. Associate it with your personal history and opinions, and you'll strengthen your memory. If you play a starring role in what you're trying to remember, you'll be more likely to remember it.

Say you're meeting Joe Blow for an interview in a hotel lobby, and you've never met him before. There's a conference at the hotel, and the lobby will be crowded with lots of guys who could be Joe Blow. So you google him and find a picture. He has brown eyes and white hair. But that's just what you see. If you leave it at that, your processing for the memory of this face will be one-dimensional, impersonal, and, well, not very memorable.

Make his face more about you to increase the likelihood that you'll recognize him when you see him in the lobby. He has a nose like your uncle Mike's. He looks a little like David Byrne from Talking Heads. "Burning Down the House" was one of your favorite songs when you were a teenager. Now you've got deeper-processing, personal associations, more cues, and oh look, there he is! Linking new information (this photo of Joe Blow) to personal information about you (your uncle Mike, David Byrne) strengthens the formation and retrieval of memories. When it comes to memory, whenever possible, make it about you.

7. LOOK FOR THE DRAMA. Emotionally charged, pulse-zapping life experiences—both good and bad—are more likely to be consolidated and are more resistant to forgetting than are emotionally neutral life events. Experiences drenched in emotion or surprise tend to be remembered—successes, humiliations, failures, weddings, births, divorces, deaths. Emotion and surprise activate your amygdala, which then sends a loud and clear message to your hippocampus: *Hey! What is going on right now is extremely important. Remember this!* And so emotion and surprise strongly facilitate the consolidation of new memories.

Events and information that elicit strong emotion also tend to matter to us, and because these events and information matter to our life narratives, we often retell these stories. And in the retelling, we are repeating and rehearsing and consequently reactivating the neural circuits, making those memories stronger.

8. MIX IT UP. Sameness is the kiss of death to memory. I can't remember the details of dinner last Tuesday because it was a typical weeknight with the kids, and those dinners suffer from a high degree of sameness—pasta, pizza, panini. Tuesday's dinner was discarded because that meal was ho-hum and our memory system isn't interested in ho-hum. I can remember dinner the night before the Oscars in February 2015 in vivid detail because that experience was momentous. No macaroni and cheese that night, thank you very much. If you want to remember more of what happened, step out of your routine.

Remember George Clooney in the red Ferrari? Look for ways to make your days and nights special, different, unusual.

9. PRACTICE MAKES PERFECT. Repetition and rehearsal strengthen memories, whether these are semantic, episodic, or muscle. For memorizing semantic information, spaced-out practice works better than cramming does, and overlearning (testing at 100 percent and then continuing to study) fortifies that memory even more. Quizzing yourself enhances your memory for the material far better than does simply rereading it.

Muscle memories become stronger and are more efficiently retrieved the more you rehearse a skill. And because these memories tell the body what to do, your body gets better at doing these physical tasks with practice.

Keeping and rereading a diary, perusing through photo albums and social media posts from years ago, and reminiscing (remember the time when?) are all ways of repeating and rehearsing episodic memories to reinforce them. But be warned. As we've learned, your episodic memories are like wide-eyed toddlers at Disney World. Your memory for what happened will probably be stronger every time you remember it, but it will also probably be altered.

10. USE PLENTY OF STRONG RETRIEVAL CUES. Cues are crucial for retrieving memories. The right cue can trigger the memory of something you haven't thought of in decades. If you want to increase your odds of recalling a particular memory, create multiple strong neural pathways that lead to its activation.

Cues can be anything associated with what you're trying to remember—the time of day, a pillbox, concert tickets on the floor by the front door, a Taylor Swift song, Cookie Monster on a talking horse, the smell of Tide laundry detergent. Smell is an especially powerful cue for evoking memory. Because your olfactory bulb (where smells are perceived—you smell in your brain, not your nose!) sends strong neural inputs to your limbic system (both the amygdala and the hippocampus), the neural architecture among smell, emotion, and memory is richly connected.

A woman steps into the elevator with you. You inhale and recognize the perfume as Obsession by Calvin Klein, and you're instantly flooded with memories of a girlfriend from college, a relationship you hadn't thought about in years.

11. BE POSITIVE. People will often tell me that they have a terrible memory. Hearing that kind of attitude, I believe them. Older adults are shown a list of negative words about aging, such as:

> decrepit,
> senile,

handicapped,
feeble.

They performed worse on memory and physical tests than did same-age subjects shown a list of positive words about aging, such as:

wise,
elder,
vibrant,
experienced.

Like people, your memory will function better if it has high self-esteem. Speak nicely to and of your memory, and it will remember more and forget less.

12. EXTERNALIZE YOUR MEMORY. People with the best memories for what they intend to do later use memory aids—lists, pillboxes, calendars, sticky notes, and other reminders. But wait. You're wondering if, and worried that, maybe you'll worsen your memory's capabilities if you rely too heavily on these external memory "crutches" instead of just using your brain. Stop worrying, and write it down.

Our prospective memory—our memory for what we intend to do later—is inherently terrible. You can try to remember that you have a dentist appointment on the first Monday of next month at 4:00, or you can enter the information in the calendar on your phone. With all we know about the high likelihood of prospective-memory failure (remember how Yo-Yo Ma forgot his precious cello in the trunk of the taxi), I strongly suggest you use your phone.

This brings me to a set of questions I hear regularly: Will using my smartphone make me dumber? If I rely on my phone to remember all my phone numbers or to google every name I can't remember, will I end up with "digital amnesia"?

Tom Gruber, an expert in artificial intelligence and cognitive science and cocreator of Siri, told me, "No. You don't lose memory by augmenting it." We're already sharing the job of memory with our smartphones in significant ways. And there's nothing wrong with doing so. "Your computer or phone is just an alternative pathway to retrieving the information you want," he says.

But if you're like me, you don't even know your own children's phone numbers. Shouldn't we? Well, we could take the time to memorize these phone numbers, but we don't need to. And not committing phone numbers to memory doesn't make us dumber. I have over two thousand phone numbers saved in the contacts list in my phone. My memory ability doesn't benefit from memorizing any of them.

Job sharing your semantic memory with Google can form a phenomenal partnership. Gruber says, "We can exponentially and infinitely expand what our brains have access to. So rather than relying on the facts and figures I learned in grade school and college, I can ask Google anything and get the information. Life is now an open-book test." And augmenting our semantic memory with information we can retrieve from Google gives us the opportunity to learn and know more.

It's the same thing with episodic memories. Two years ago, I went to Venice with Joe. I don't remember the name of the hotel we stayed in, the restaurant where we ate with my friend Kathlene, the name of the amazing bottle of wine we shared, or the name of the place where we rented kayaks. But because I took photos that recorded my geolocation and I posted some of these photos to Instagram with captions describing what we did, and because I stored the name of the hotel in my calendar, my smartphone can help me piece together the episodic memories of this trip in vivid and accurate detail.

So don't be afraid of sharing the job of memory with technology. You don't think twice about augmenting your vision with eyeglasses. So why not your memory? Even a great memory isn't perfect. Memories augmented by our phones are usually more reliable than what we can retrieve if left to our own devices (pun intended).

13. CONTEXT MATTERS. Memory retrieval is far easier, faster, and more likely to be fully remembered when the internal and external conditions match whatever they were

when that memory was formed. As we saw with the deep-sea divers who learned underwater or on the beach, your learning circumstances matter. If you drink mocha Frappuccinos while studying for a test, have another one when you take the exam.

14. CHILL OUT. Most of us are regularly stressed out, and chronic stress is nothing but bad news for our ability to remember. In addition to making you more vulnerable to a whole host of diseases, chronic stress impairs memory and shrinks your hippocampus. While we can't necessarily free ourselves from the stress in our lives, we can change how we react to it. Through yoga, meditation, exercise, and practices in mindfulness, gratitude, and compassion, we can train our brains to become less reactive, to put the brakes on the runaway stress response, and to stay healthy in the face of chronic, toxic stress.

15. GET ENOUGH SLEEP. You need seven to nine hours of nightly slumber to optimally consolidate the new memories you created today. Sleep is critical for locking into long-term memory whatever you have learned and experienced. If you don't get enough sleep, you'll go through the next day experiencing a form of amnesia. Some of your memories from yesterday might be fuzzy, inaccurate, or even missing. And you've just increased your amyloid levels. Getting enough sleep reduces your risk of developing Alzheimer's.

16. WHEN TRYING TO REMEMBER SOMEONE'S NAME, TURN YOUR Bakers INTO bakers. Can you remember what that means?

Suggested Reading

Baddeley, A. *Working Memory*. Oxford, U.K.: Clarendon, 1986.

———. "Working Memory, Theories Models and Controversy." *Annual Review of Psychology* 63 (2012): 12.1–12.29.

Baddeley, A., M. W. Eysenck, and M. C. Anderson. *Memory*. 2nd ed. New York: Psychology Press, 2015.

Bjork, R. A., and A. E. Woodward. "Directed Forgetting of Individual Words in Free Recall." *Journal of Experimental Psychology* 99 (1973): 22–27.

Blake, A. B., M. Nazarian, and A. D. Castel. "The Apple of the Mind's Eye: Everyday Attention, Metamemory, and Reconstructive Memory of the Apple Logo." *Quarterly Journal of Experimental Psychology* 68 (2015): 858–865.

Brown, J. "Some Tests of the Decay Theory of Immediate Memory." *Quarterly Journal of Experimental Psychology* 10, no. 1 (1958): 12–21.

Butler, A. C., and H. L. Roediger III. "Testing Improves Long-Term Retention in a Simulated Classroom Setting." *European Journal of Cognitive Psychology* 19 (2007): 514–527.

Charles, S. T., M. Mather, and L. L. Carstersen, "Aging and Emotional Memory: The Forgettable Nature of Negative Images for Older Adults." *Journal of Experimental Psychology: General* 132, no. 1. (2003): 310–324.

Corkin, S. "What's New with Amnesic Patient HM?" *Nature Reviews Neuroscience* 3 (2002): 153–160.

———. *Permanent Present Tense: The Unforgettable Life of the Amnesiac Patient, H.M.* New York: Basic Books, 2013.

Dittrich, L. *Patient H.M.: A Story of Memory, Madness, and Family Secrets*. New York: Random House, 2016.

Ebbinghaus, H. *Memory: A Contribution to Experimental Psychology*. New York: Dover Publications, 1885; reprint 1964.

Eich, E. "Memory for Unattended Events: Remembering With and Without Awareness." *Memory & Cognition* 12 (1984): 105–111.

Eichenbaum, H. *The Cognitive Neuroscience of Memory: An Introduction*. 2nd ed. New York: Oxford University Press, 2012.

Foer, J. *Moonwalking with Einstein: The Art and Science of Remembering Everything*. New York: Penguin Books, 2011.

Godden, D. R., and A. D. Baddeley. "Context-Dependent Memory in Two Natural Environments: On Land and Under Water." *British Journal of Psychology* 66 (1975): 325–331.

Gothe, K., K. Oberauer, and R. Kliegl. "Age Differences in Dual-Task Performance After Practice." *Psychology and Aging* 22 (2007): 596–606.

Henner, M. *Total Memory Makeover: Uncover Your Past, Take Charge of Your Future.* New York: Gallery Books, 2013.

Hirst, W., E. A. Phelps, R. L. Buckner, A. E. Budson, A. Cuc, J. D. E. Gabrieli, and M. K. Johnson. "Long-Term Memory for the Terrorist Attack of September 11: Flashbulb Memories, Event Memories, and the Factors That Influence Their Retention." *Journal of Experimental Psychology: General* 138 (2009): 161–176.

Hirst, W., E. A. Phelps, R. Meksin, C. J. Vaidya, M. K. Johnson, K. J. Mitchell, and A. Olsson. "A Ten-Year Follow-Up of a Study of Memory for the Attack of September 11, 2001: Flashbulb Memories and Memories for Flashbulb Events." *Journal of Experimental Psychology: General* 144 (2015): 604–623.

Holzel, B., J. Carmody, M. Vangel, C. Congleton, S. M. Yerramsetti, T. Gard, and S. W. Lazar. "Mindfulness Practice Leads to Increases in Regional Brain Gray Matter Density." *Psychiatry Research* 191 (2011): 36–43.

Isaacson, R. S., C. A. Ganzer, H. Hristov, K. Hackett, E. Caesar, R. Cohen, et al. "The Clinical Practice of Risk Reduction for Alzheimer's Disease: A Precision Medicine Approach." *Alzheimer's & Dementia.* 12 (2018): 1663–1673.

Johansson, L., X. Guo, M. Waern, S. Östling, D. Gustafson, C. Bengtsson, and I. Skoog. "Midlife Psychological Stress and Risk of Dementia: A 35-Year Longitudinal Population Study." *Brain* 133 (2010): 2,217–2,224.

Karpicke, J. D., and H. L. Roediger. "The Critical Importance of Retrieval for Learning." *Science* 319 (2008): 966–968.

Kivipelto M. A. Solomon, S. Ahtiluoto, T. Ngandu, J. Lehtisalo, R. Antikainen, et al. "The Finnish Geriatric Intervention Study to Prevent Cognitive Impairment and Disability (FINGER): Study Design and Progress." *Alzheimer's & Dementia*. 9 (2013): 657–665.

Loftus, E. F. "Reconstructing Memory: The Incredible Eyewitness." *Psychology Today* 8 (1974): 116–119.

———. "When a Lie Becomes a Memory's Truth: Memory Distortion After Exposure to Misinformation." *Current Directions in Psychological Science* 1 (1992): 121–123.

Loftus, E. F., and J. C. Palmer. "Reconstruction of Automobile Destruction: An Example of the Interaction Between Language and Memory." *Journal of Verbal Learning and Verbal Behavior* 13 (1974): 585–589.

Loftus, E. F., and G. Zanni. "Eyewitness Testimony: The Influence of the Wording of a Question." *Bulletin of the Psychonomic Society* 5 (1975): 86–88.

Loftus, E. F., and J. E. Pickrell. "The Formation of False Memories." *Psychiatric Annals* 25 (1995): 720–725.

MacKay, D. G. *Remembering: What 50 Years of Research with Famous Amnesia Patient H.M. Can Teach Us about Memory and How It Works.* Amherst, NY: Prometheus Books, 2019.

Mantyla, T., and L. G. Nilsson. "Remembering to Remember in Adulthood: A Population-Based Study on Aging and Prospective Memory." *Aging, Neuropsychology, and Cognition* 4 (1997): 81–92.

McDaniel, M. A., and G. O. Einstein. *Prospective Memory: An Overview and Synthesis of an Emerging Field.* Thousand Oaks, CA: Sage, 2007.

McGaugh, J. L. *Memory and Emotion: The Making of Lasting Memories.* New York: Columbia University Press, 2003.

Melby-Lervag, M., and C. Hulme. "There Is No Convincing Evidence That Working Memory Training Is Effective." *Psychonomic Bulletin & Review* 23 (2015): 324–330.

Miller, G. A. "The Magical Number Is Seven, Plus or Minus Two: Some Limits on Our Capacity for Processing Information." *Psychological Review* 63 (1956): 81–97.

Neupert, S. D., T. R. Patterson, A. A. Davis, and J. C. Allaire. "Age Differences in Daily Predictors of Forgetting to Take Medication: The Importance of Context and Cognition." *Experimental Aging Research* 37 (2011): 435–448.

Nickerson, R. S., and J. J. Adams. "Long-Term Memory for a Common Object." *Cognitive Psychology* 11 (1979): 287–307.

O'Brien, G. *On Pluto: Inside the Mind of Alzheimer's.* Canada: Codfish Press. 2018.

O'Kane, G., E. A. Kensinger, and S. Corkin. "Evidence for Semantic Learning in Profound Amnesia: An Investigation with H.M." *Hippocampus* 14 (2004): 417–425.

Patihis, L., and E. G. Loftus. "Crashing Memory 2.0: False Memories in Adults for an Upsetting Childhood Event." *Applied Cognitive Psychology* 31 (2016): 41–50.

Peterson, L. R., and M. J. Peterson. "Short-Term Retention of Individual Verbal Items." *Journal of Experimental Psychology* 58, no. 3 (1959): 193–198.

Pink, D. H. *When: The Scientific Secrets of Perfect Timing.* New York: Riverhead Books, 2018.

Reisberg, D., and P. Hertel. *Memory and Emotion.* New York: Oxford University Press, 2004.

Salthouse, T. A. "The Processing-Speed Theory of Adult Age Differences in Cognition." *Psychological Review* 103 (1996): 403–428.

———. "Attempted Decomposition of Age-Related Influences on Two Tests of Reasoning." *Psychology and Aging* 16 (2001): 251–263.

———. "Perspectives on Aging." *Psychological Science* 1 (2006): 68–87.

Salthouse, T. A., D. E. Berish, and J. D. Miles. "The Role of Cognitive Stimulation on the Relations Between Age and Cognitive Functioning." *Psychology and Aging* 17 (2002): 548–557.

Schacter, D. L. *The Seven Sins of Memory: How the Mind Forgets and Remembers.* New York: Houghton-Mifflin, 2001.

Schmolck, H., A. W. Buffalo, and L. R. Squire. "Memory Distortions Develop over Time: Recollections of the O. J. Simpson Verdict After 15 and 32 Months." *Psychological Science* 11 (2000): 39–45.

Schwartz, B. L. *Memory: Foundations and Applications.* Thousand Oaks, CA: Sage Publications, 2018.

Schwartz, B. L., and L. D. Frazier. "Tip-of-the-Tongue States and Aging: Contrasting Psycholinguistic and Metacognitive Perspectives." *Journal of General Psychology* 132 (2005): 377–391.

Schwartz, B. L., and J. Metcalfe. "Tip-of-the-Tongue (TOT) States: Retrieval, Behavior, and Experience." *Memory and Cognition* 39 (2011): 737–749.

Sedikides, C., and J. D. Green. "Memory As a Self-Protective Mechanism." *Social and Personality Psychology Compass* 3, no. 6 (2009): 1,055–1,068.

Shaw, J. *The Memory Illusion: Remembering, Forgetting, and the Science of False Memory.* New York: Random House, 2016.

Slotnick, S. D. *Cognitive Neuroscience of Memory.* New York: Cambridge University Press, 2017.

Snowdon, D. A. "Healthy Aging and Dementia: Findings from the Nun Study." *Annals of Internal Medicine* 139 (2003): 450–454.

Squire, L. R., and E. R. Kandel. *Memory: From Mind to Molecules.* Greenwood Village, CO: Roberts & Co., 2009.

Walker, M. P. *Why We Sleep: Unlocking the Power of Sleep and Dreams.* New York: Scribner, 2017.

Walker, M. P., and R. Stickgold, "Sleep-Dependent Learning and Memory Consolidation." *Neuron* 44 (2004): 121–123.

Wilson, R. S., D. A. Evans, J. L. Bienias, C. F. Mendes de Leon, J. A. Schneider, and D. A. Bennett. "Proneness to Psychological Distress Is Associated with Risk of Alzheimer's Disease." *Neurology* 6 (2003): 1,479–1,485.

Winograd, E., and U. Neisser. *Affect and Accuracy in Recall: Studies of "Flashbulb" Memories.* Emory Symposia in Cognition. New York: Cambridge University Press, 1992.

Acknowledgments

Many thanks to everyone who helped bring *Remember* to fruition. Thank you to Jennifer Rudolph Walsh for championing me and this book and thanks to Suzanne Gluck for so enthusiastically picking up that baton. Thank you to Gina Centrello for believing in this project and giving me a home at Random House. Thanks to Tammy Blake, Patricia Boyd, Marnie Cochran, Danielle Curtis, Brianne Sperber, Melissa Sanford, Christina Foxley, and the entire Random House team, and especially to my editor, Diana Baroni, for pushing me to find the best version of this book.

Thank you to Dr. John Kelsey, professor emeritus of psychology at Bates College, for editing a draft and keeping me honest with every word. It was such a treat to work with you again. Thanks to my dear friend Dr. Edward Meloni, assistant professor of psychiatry at Harvard Medical School, for your insights into the current understanding of PTSD and memory.

Thank you to Marilu Henner for your friendship and many fascinating conversations about living with highly superior autobiographical memory. Thanks to Tom Gruber for taking the time to talk with me about artificial intelligence, human memory, and the benefits of sharing the job of memory with external technology. Thank you to Joshua Foer for chatting with me about his experience as a memory champion and the pros and cons of using memory techniques in everyday life. Thanks to Roberto Borgatti for explaining the steps for learning to swing a golf club. Thank you to my dear friend Greg O'Brien for sharing so candidly what it feels like to forget because of Alzheimer's. You are my hero.

Lastly, thanks and so much love to my dedicated cast of early readers: Anne Carey, Laurel Daly, Joe Deitch, Mary Genova, Tom Genova, Kim Howland, and Mary MacGregor. This was great fun!

About the Author

Lisa Genova is the *New York Times* bestselling author of the novels *Still Alice*, *Left Neglected*, *Love Anthony*, *Inside the O'Briens*, and *Every Note Played*. *Still Alice* was adapted into an Oscar-winning film starring Julianne Moore, Alec Baldwin, and Kristen Stewart. Lisa graduated valedictorian from Bates College with a degree in biopsychology and holds a PhD in neuroscience from Harvard University. She travels worldwide speaking about the neurological diseases she writes about and has appeared on *The Dr. Oz Show*, *Today*, *PBS NewsHour*, CNN, and NPR. Her TED talk, "What You Can Do to Prevent Alzheimer's," has been viewed more than five million times.